Essential Stress Reduction Workbook for Teens

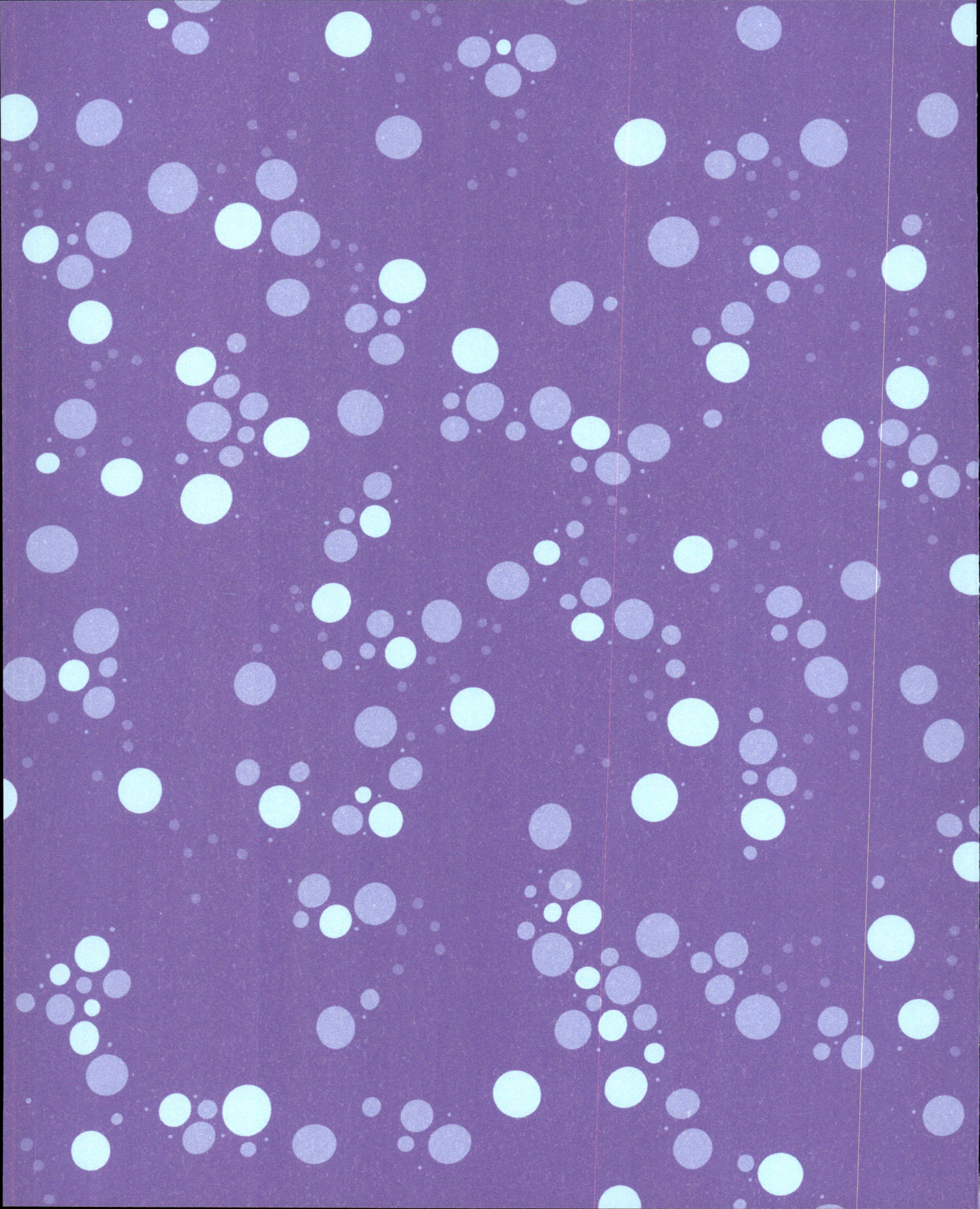

Essential Stress Reduction Workbook for Teens

CBT and Mindfulness Tools to Soothe Stress and Cultivate Calm

Dr. Carla Cirilli Andrews, PsyD

Illustrations by Tara O'Brien

R

ROCKRIDGE
PRESS

Interior and Cover Designer: Stephanie Mautone
Art Producer: Samantha Ulban
Editor: Jesse Aylen
Production Editor: Andrew Yackira
Illustrations © 2020 Tara O'Brien

ISBN: Print 978-1-64876-095-2 | eBook 978-1-64876-096-9
R0

To my parents and sisters, for loving me through those difficult teen years, and my husband and daughter, who are my peace in a stressful world.

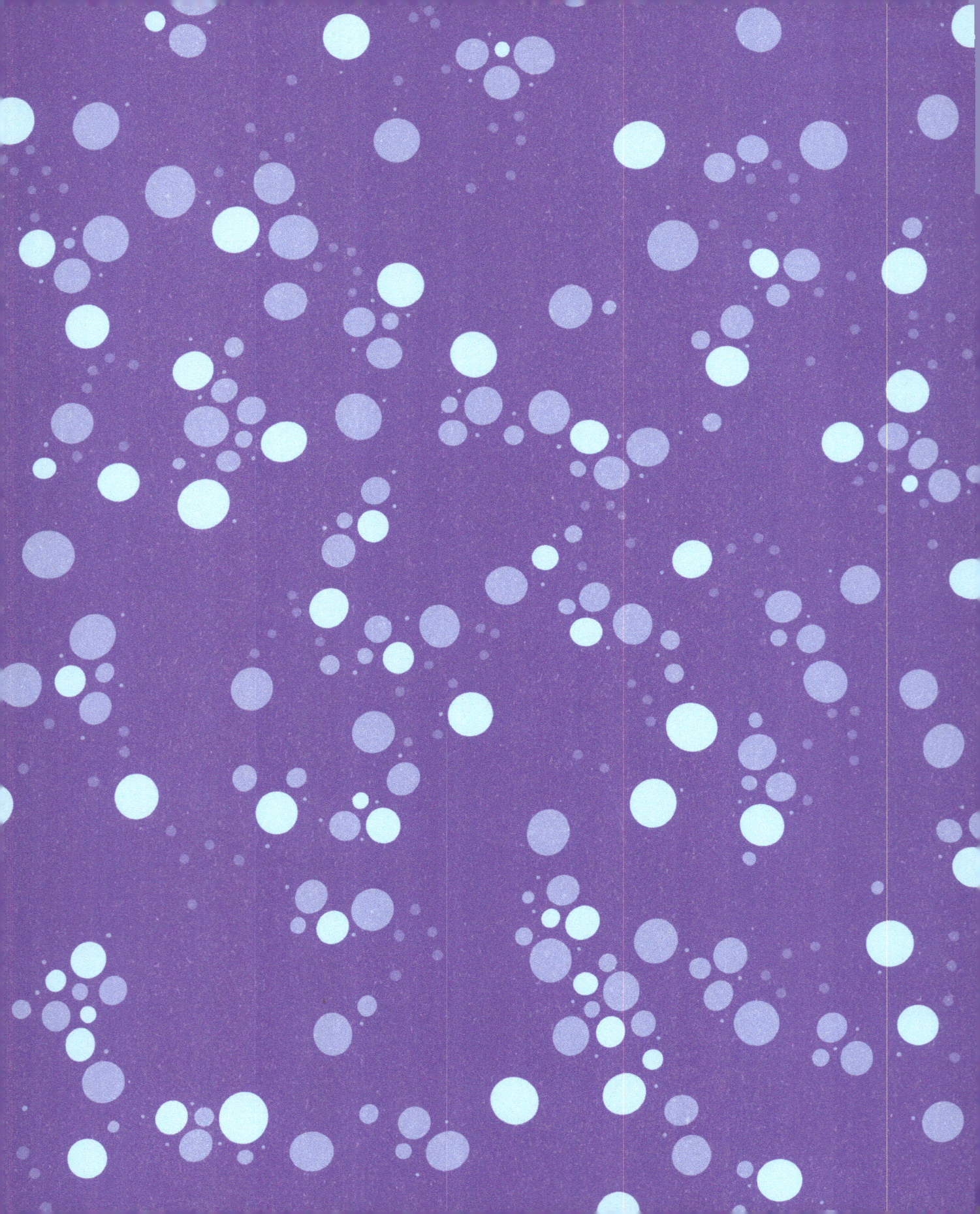

Contents

Introduction

Dear Reader,

I am so glad you're reading this workbook! Either you're a teen who's decided to better manage your stress, or you care about a teen who is negatively affected by stress. Either way, this workbook is a comprehensive yet practical guide to managing stress. My hope is that each teen who comes across this book feels empowered to conquer any stressor that arises in their daily life using the accessible, everyday tools and techniques we'll be exploring together.

I'm a licensed clinical psychologist, and I specialize in counseling teens through the transition from childhood to adulthood. In the safe space of the therapy room, I often hear "I feel like I'm the only one struggling . . . it seems like everyone else has it all figured out." In reality, many teens, including the ones I see in my practice, are experiencing similar pressures: balancing schoolwork, competitiveness, social media pressures, uncertainty about the future, and maintaining relationships with family and friends. It's not easy! And if this sounds familiar, know that you are not alone.

I'm here to tell you that *everyone* experiences stress in daily life—the difference is how we choose to respond to it. While you can't control the world around you, you *can* control how you react. I teach the same stress-management techniques to different teens, and hear from those teens and their parents that they feel happier, calmer, and more in control of their lives. I hope this book can have the same positive effect on each and every person who reads and works with it.

The goal of this workbook is *not* to eliminate stress altogether. At a basic level, stress is natural and can be helpful in some situations. The goal, instead, is to learn how to manage stress in a healthy way that challenges us and helps us grow. Think of this workbook as a general guide to inform your personal journey. Along the way, I'll share the knowledge and strategies you need to move forward. You will become more prepared as you successfully navigate each task. Ultimately, you will master the skills you need to have a happier, calmer life. Here's a quick overview of the journey:

- Part 1 will cover the basics about stress. You'll gain knowledge by finding answers to common questions like: *What is stress exactly? Is it different from anxiety? What are the basic stress-reducing techniques I need to know?*

- Part 2 will present exercises to help you learn and practice new skills in a way that's individually suited to you. I'll share the techniques that I use in therapy, and you'll complete short activities that personalize these skills for you.

- Part 3 will present real-life situations that teens often describe as stressful. In a question-and-answer format, I'll offer guidance on navigating them by applying the knowledge and skills covered in parts 1 and 2.

Now that we have a clear picture of the journey ahead, let's get started!

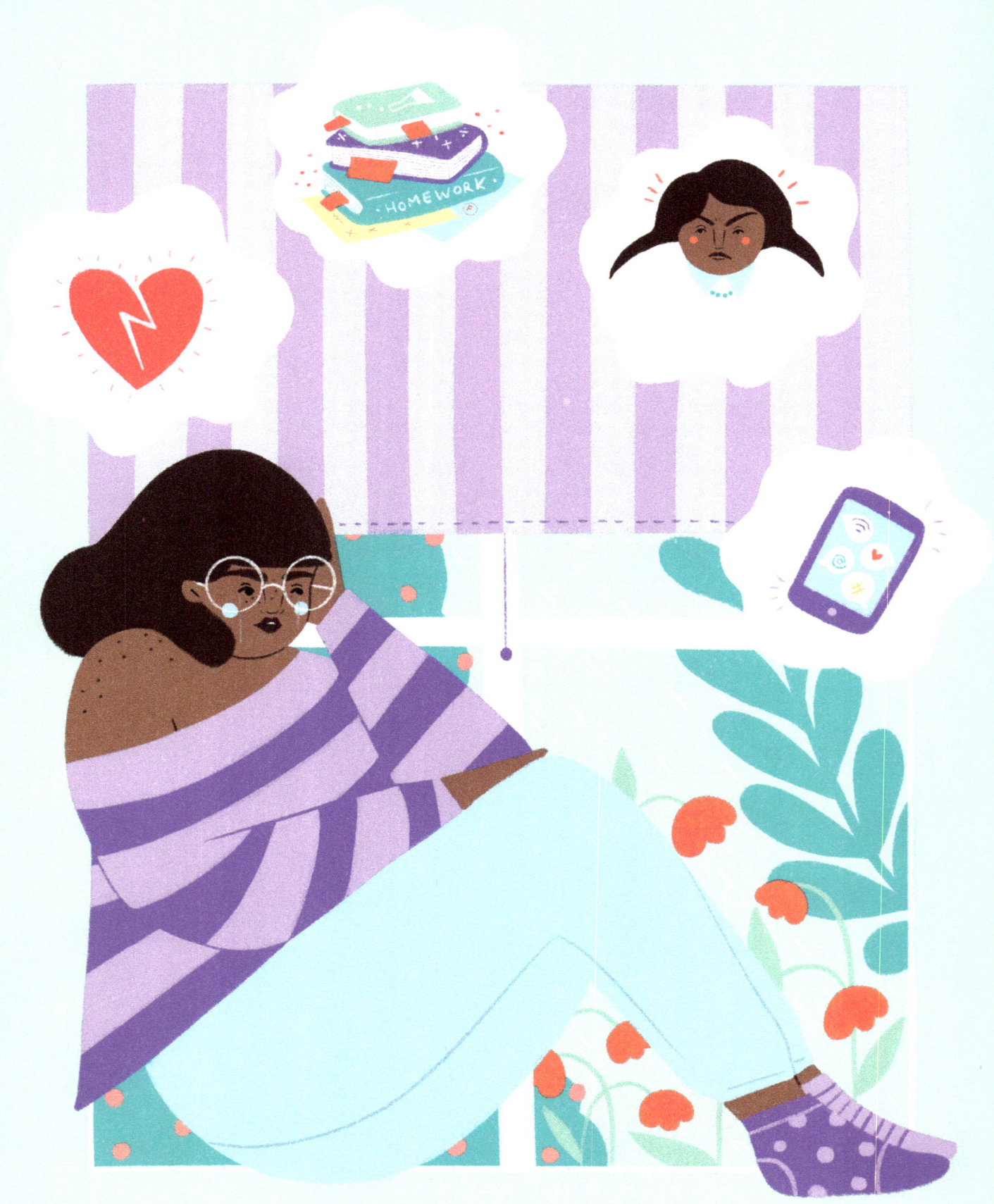

PART 1

The Scoop on Stress

Before we can learn to manage stress, we first have to understand it. Stress can affect us physically, mentally, and psychologically, so together we'll take a closer look at each of these areas. Once you have a solid foundation about exactly what stress is and how it specifically affects you, the path to effective stress reduction will become a lot clearer. After learning a variety of techniques that are proven to reduce stress, you'll be encouraged to try all of them and decide which techniques work best for you.

continued ▶

WHAT DOES IT MEAN TO BE STRESSED?

"I'm stressed out" is a common phrase, but what exactly does it mean? Very simply, stress is a natural response that we develop when we face a challenge. This may happen when our bodies respond to a physical challenge like pushing yourself to finish a race, or when our minds respond to a mental challenge like cramming the night before a test. Additionally, psychological or emotional challenges can cause us stress, such as an unexpected or painful romantic breakup, or a fight with our siblings or parents. Very often a stressor can affect us physically, mentally, *and* psychologically. Imagine midterms week at school: You may get very little sleep or skip meals, you probably hold marathon study sessions, and you may constantly worry about grades. During this stressful week, your body, mind, and emotions are all pushed to the point of exhaustion.

Although we can't eliminate life stressors like exams, we can certainly learn new techniques to manage them. Daily stressors, small and large, will continue to arise, but they don't have to hold you back from success or stop you from doing things you love. In fact, learning how to handle stress can actually empower you to be more resilient, making you more able to recover quickly from difficult challenges. You might think of resilience as a "superpower," because it helps you bounce back from any setback. Again, the goal of this workbook is not to eliminate stress entirely. The goal is to build up your resilience "superpower" so that you can effectively cope, adapt, and persevere. A small amount of stress can sometimes be helpful by providing the attention and energy we need to overcome everyday challenges. Let's turn now to some facts about exactly how stress affects our brains and our bodies in both positive and negative ways.

THE IMMEDIATE EFFECTS ON YOUR BRAIN

What happens to our brain when we confront a stressful situation? Our brains are excellent at recognizing danger around us and responding immediately. After all, we need a rapid and reliable response to keep us safe in emergency situations. If you smell smoke and see flames, your brain instantly determines that there's a fire and prepares your body to run away. Our brains and bodies are constantly communicating back and forth. First, your body (your nose) alerts your brain to the smell of smoke, then your brain sends an emergency signal (stress hormones) back to your body (leg muscles), carrying you to safety. Sometimes this response to stress is absolutely necessary!

That instantaneous response can be helpful on a daily basis, too. Here's just one example of a particularly stressful morning showing how beneficial stress can be in the smallest of ways:

First thing on a Monday morning, I roll over in bed to glance at the clock and realize I slept through my alarm. Aaaah! My brain suddenly releases a jolt of energy. I hop out of bed and get ready in record time. Still, I'm running late for school! Thankfully, my brain supplies a steady amount of energy to help me rush to my first class. I make it to my seat in time . . . only to remember that I'm supposed to give a presentation today. Can this morning get any worse?! As it gets closer to my turn to present, I feel a rush of nerves. Wow—this shot of energy actually improves my attention and focus and helps me deliver a pretty good presentation even on the fly. Nice! Once it's over, I settle into my seat and notice an instant feeling of calm as the stress passes.

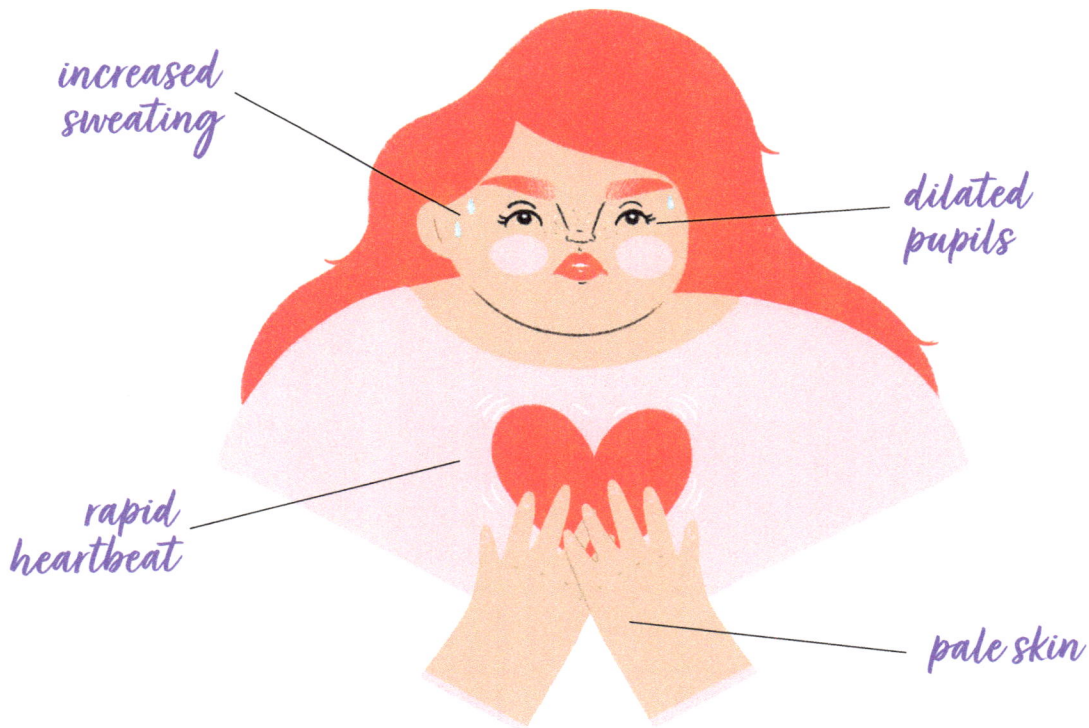

increased sweating

dilated pupils

rapid heartbeat

pale skin

The basic science at work during this stressful morning is the fight-or-flight response. Remember, our brains are constantly scanning the environment for potential dangers of all shapes and sizes. The thought of failing your presentation counts as a threat. In response, your brain releases stress hormones, like cortisol, just as if there were a true emergency like a fire. Our bodies then prepare for "fight or flight": either your body gears up to confront the threat, or you try to escape it. In either case, your heart starts racing, your breathing quickens, your muscles tighten or tremble, and you may feel hot and flushed. Your mind will find it hard to concentrate on anything but that one stressor, and emotions may overwhelm you.

The target, then, is *just the right amount of stress response* for *just the right amount of time*. During that stressful morning, you can see how a moderate amount of stress for an hour or two was tolerable and even helpful. But if you felt too much stress about that presentation, you might panic and experience stage fright. If you felt too little stress, it would take away your motivation to work hard; after all, if you don't care about your grade, you won't put in much effort. But experiencing a moderate amount of stress for a short amount of time can actually help you succeed. Other examples include using nervous energy about an upcoming exam to motivate a productive study session, turning nerves into excitement when asking someone on a date, or overcoming the fear of losing a big sporting match by bringing your A game.

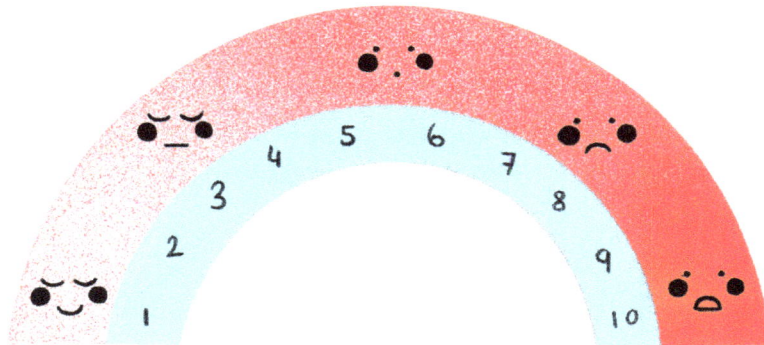

Can you think of a time when a moderate amount of stress actually helped you succeed in some way?

_____

_____

_____

_____

_____

_____

Chronic Stress and Stress Overload

But of course, there's a flip side. If you experience *too much stress* for *too long*, your brain starts to release more stress hormones for an extended amount of time, as if you are stuck in "fight or flight." When that happens, you may notice that you're:

- unable to focus

- forgetful and disorganized

- constantly worrying

- more emotional than usual

- irritable or quick to react to small triggers

- suffering from a pessimistic outlook or depression

If you feel that this is happening to you right now, it's important to speak to a parent, caregiver, therapist, and/or doctor. Think of it as a team approach; while you are the star player in managing your response to stressors, asking for help from your teammates can help you reach your goal as soon as possible.

A lot of teens wonder how to "shut off" their brain's stress response, but as we've seen, we should appreciate that our brains are at work 24/7. The techniques offered in this workbook are meant to give you more control over your thoughts, feelings, and reactions so that you can achieve *just the right amount of stress* for *just the right amount of time.*

The Effects on Your Body

Now that you have a good understanding of how stress affects your brain, let's turn our attention to how stress affects your body and behaviors. If you experience *too much stress* for *too long*, your brain gets stuck in "fight-or-flight" mode, meaning your body is constantly prepared for action. It becomes difficult to relax because you always feel tense and unsettled. If you remember, your brain releases stress hormones like cortisol in short spurts to energize you when needed. If a lot of cortisol is released over a long period of time, it can negatively affect your heart, digestive system, and immune system, making you more prone to illness and chronic medical conditions.

While it can be hard to see these long-term changes to your health, you may notice smaller physical symptoms (such as headaches, stomachaches, or diarrhea) or changes in your day-to-day behaviors like:

- trouble sleeping

- changes in eating (eating more or less than usual)

- nervous habits (nail-biting, fidgeting)
- increased use of drugs, vaping, or alcohol in order to relax
- avoiding activities that make you feel nervous

Can you think of how your own body responds to stress?

_____

_____

_____

_____

_____

_____

Is It Stress or Anxiety?

You may wonder what the difference is between feeling *stressed* and feeling *anxious*. We defined *stress* as our body's natural response in the face of a challenge, which can affect us physically, mentally, and psychologically. We also learned that when a stressful event happens, our brains react with a "fight-or-flight" response. *Anxiety* is the word used to describe the emotional reaction that we feel during these times. Remember our high-stress example of midterms week? Your brain's *stress* response might cause trouble sleeping, loss of appetite, lack of focus, and stomachaches. Your *anxiety* may feel like constant worry about your grades, nervousness all week long, and that racing heartbeat you notice as you start each exam.

With typical day-to-day stress, two things usually happen: We figure out a pretty good way to cope with it temporarily, and then we feel better as time passes. Or, anxiety overloads our ability to cope, and it might last for a longer time. When anxious feelings overwhelm a person every day for several months, this can create problems with their health, mood, relationships, schoolwork, or employment. These may be signs of an anxiety disorder, which is important to discuss with parents, caregivers, a doctor, or a therapist. The good news is, the techniques you learn in this book can be used to reduce both stress and anxiety.

Reaching Out for a Helping Hand

Everybody needs help sometimes, but it can feel hard to ask for it. Teens can feel like they want to—or should know how to—solve their own problems. It's as if asking for help is a sign of weakness. In reality, it takes a lot of courage to be honest with yourself and with others when you're having a hard time.

Help and support from other people can come in different forms, like simply sharing your feelings, asking for advice, brainstorming solutions to a problem together, or getting sympathy and emotional support from others.

Everyone needs support, and mixing and matching different types of help from various people might be just the answer you're looking for. You may have one trusted friend you can confide in, and another friend who you can depend on for a good laugh. One caring adult may listen with a sympathetic ear, while another offers a joke to lift your mood paired with some great advice. We'll also discuss asking for help in more detail in activity 14 (page 49).

If you find that your social network (friends, family, teachers, coaches, community leaders) isn't meeting your needs, it can be helpful to talk to a professional therapist (counselor, social worker, psychologist, or psychiatrist). Therapy doesn't have to be a lifelong commitment; often, teens just need a safe space for a little while to fully open up. You can ask a parent, a teacher, a school counselor, or your doctor about finding a local therapist. The end of this workbook includes two resource sections for more information. If at any time you feel you are a danger to yourself or others, including self-harming or thinking about suicide, please skip to the Crisis Resources section (page 123) now to find options for immediate support.

10 STRATEGIES TO TRY TODAY

The following techniques—proven to reduce stress—can be used in two ways. First, you can call on them to help instantly calm you down when you notice stress overload. Second, you can add them into your routine to manage the smaller stressors that build up over time and can eventually lead to stress overload. This bit-by-bit way of preventing stress overload is proven by research; for example, practicing meditation can actually reduce the amount of cortisol your brain releases into your body. They might not seem like it at first, but these are powerful tactics in your quest to conquer stress.

These strategies are presented as a menu for you to explore, to sample, and to select what works for you. You may find that one or two strategies always make you feel better, while some work better in certain situations, and others might not work at all. I trust that you will know what works best for you, but I also ask that you try every single strategy at least once. Keep an open mind; a brand-new technique might do the trick. For best results, practice these strategies on a regular basis when you are feeling fine, so that they become a habit you can rely on when you're under stress. Along the way, you will notice your "stress reduction backpack" stocking up with more and more helpful tools for conquering any stress that crosses your path.

Before you try these 10 strategies, take a moment to check in with your body and mind right now. Do you notice any stress? Are your muscles tense? Do you have worried thoughts crossing your mind? As you try these 10 strategies, take note of any calming effect they might have.

Deep Breathing

Deep breathing is a simple but effective technique that can quiet both the mind and the body. Increasing the supply of oxygen to your brain deactivates the fight-or-flight response, creating an immediate sense of calm. The best part is, you can engage in deep breathing anywhere at any time. Here's how:

- Get as comfortable as you can and close your eyes if you want.

- Take a deep breath in through your nose. Focus on the fresh air entering your body, count slowly, or imagine inhaling a calm, peaceful color traveling through your body.

- Fill your belly with air, not just your chest. Rest a hand on your stomach to sense your belly rising with your inhale.

- Exhale through your mouth, for the same amount of time or longer than the inhale. Focus on the air leaving your body, count slowly, or imagine exhaling a toxic color.

- Repeat as many times as necessary until you notice your mind is clearer and your body is calmer.

Mindfulness

Mindfulness is a practice that allows you to access a state of calm by drawing your focus to the present moment. It encourages you to let go of focusing on the past, which can lead to depressed feelings, and to stop worrying about the future, which can lead to anxious feelings. A quick, effective way to practice mindfulness is to ground yourself by focusing on your five senses. Take a moment right now to notice:

- **Sight:** What do you see around you?

- **Hearing:** What can you hear?

- **Touch:** Scan your body. What sensations do you notice in your body?

- **Smell:** Do you notice any scents around you?

- **Taste:** Do you notice any tastes in your mouth?

On a day-to-day basis, you can check in with your surroundings at any time, or you can create pleasant experiences for your five senses. For instance, look at a favorite picture, listen to a favorite song, hold an object that is soothing to touch, smell a lotion, candle, or incense that relaxes you (lavender has been shown to increase calm), or chew on a favorite mint or gum to create a pleasing taste. The secret is to focus on each sensory experience, rooting you in the present moment, and distracting your thoughts from whatever is stressing you out.

Meditation

While mindfulness is drawing your focus to one thing, meditation can be thought of as drawing your attention to nothing. The idea is to clear your mind of all thoughts, good and bad, and just enjoy stillness. Meditation is proven to reduce cortisol, thereby reducing your experience of stress. There are many types of meditation; in fact, deep breathing and mindfulness can be considered subtypes of meditation. But the idea is always to let go of the thoughts that continuously pop up in your mind. Here's a starting point:

- Get comfortable in a quiet place.

- Close your eyes or stare at a fixed object.

- Clear your mind of all thoughts, feelings, observations, and so on. It can be helpful to imagine you're painting a wall of white (or any preferred color) in your mind.

- Thoughts will pop up. Simply let each thought pass by (as if it's floating by in a bubble or like clouds in the sky) or you can mentally swipe the thought away and return to your stillness.

- You can try it for just a few seconds at first and gradually extend the amount of time you clear your mind each day.

Visualization

Visualization is a variation of mindfulness and meditation that involves imagining your "happy place," or listening to guided imagery that helps you paint a mental picture. Use your imagination to create your own personal scene that is perfectly relaxing to you. While one person might imagine a beach scene, another might picture fishing on a lake, and another might focus on their favorite memory of a roller coaster. Just like with mindfulness, use your five senses to paint the scene. Let's say you're imagining a beach scene that might include:

- **Sight:** Imagine a beautiful sunset over the horizon.

- **Hearing:** Listen to the waves move to and from the shore.

- **Touch:** Feel the warm sand under your feet.

- **Smell:** Notice the smell of the salty beach air.

- **Taste:** Imagine sipping on a refreshing lemonade and tasting salty ocean water on your lips.

Movement

While movement can include exercise, really any physical activity can be helpful in counteracting stress by reducing levels of cortisol and increasing levels of endorphins (the brain's "feel-good" chemical). Activity with repetitive movements can be especially helpful for both the mind and body, such as:

- Walking
- Jogging/Running
- Swimming
- Biking
- Dancing
- Yoga
- Tai Chi

While some of us already have regular exercise we enjoy, others don't. In that case, start by trying any movement that is pleasurable for you—a five-minute dance break from studying could be a fun start—and try to partner up with a family member or friend to help you do it consistently.

Progressive Muscle Relaxation (PMR)

Progressive muscle relaxation is another strategy that can help calm both the body and mind. When using progressive muscle relaxation, you tense a group of muscles for 10 seconds as you breathe in, and you relax them as you breathe out. Focus on one muscle group at a time, progressing from head to toe (or vice versa). Notice the sensation of tension, and then the release of relaxation. PMR is proven to increase oxygen supply to the brain, reduce cortisol, and create a sense of calm throughout your whole body. Here's one sample PMR script, focusing on key muscle groups that often hold tension:

- **Forehead:** Raise your eyebrows and wrinkle your forehead. Hold, then release.

- **Eyes:** Close your eyes tightly and squeeze. Hold, then release.

- **Mouth:** Tense your mouth by squeezing your lips and pushing your tongue against the roof of your mouth. Hold, then release.

- **Jaws:** Clench your jaws as tightly as you can. Hold, then release.

- **Neck and shoulders:** Raise your shoulders up toward your ears and tighten your neck muscles. Hold, then release.

- **Hands:** Tighten your hands into fists and squeeze. Hold, then release.

- **Abdomen:** Tighten your stomach muscles and squeeze. Hold, then release.

- **Butt and thighs:** Tighten your buttocks and thigh muscles. Hold, then release.

- **Feet:** Tense the muscles in both feet and squeeze. Hold, then release.

Autogenic Relaxation

Like PMR, autogenic relaxation involves relaxing each muscle group one at a time, but there is an added focus on heaviness and warmth, with hypnosis-inducing repetition. Use the same PMR script, but this time repeat the following statement to yourself for each muscle group: "My [arms] are heavy and warm. My [arms] are completely calm." Once you've repeated this statement for each muscle group, add the following focus:

- "My heartbeat is calm and regular. I am completely calm."

- "My breathing is calm and regular. I am completely calm."

Mantra

A personal mantra is a statement that is meaningful and calming to you. Simply thinking of your mantra, writing it down, or saying it aloud in stressful moments can help focus your mental energy and improve your mood. To create your own mantra:

- Keep it short and memorable.

- Use the present tense.

- Repeat it frequently throughout the day (first thing in the morning and at bedtime are powerful times to focus on your mantra).

- Pick one, two, or three mantras max, that can be used in various situations to boost your own confidence and self-love. (For example: *Every problem has a solution; I control my emotions, they don't control me; I am doing my best and learning to do better; Focus on the good.*)

Gratitude Practice

Another simple yet productive way to quickly reduce stress is to shift your perspective. When you're under stress, it is easy to focus on everything that is going wrong. Practicing gratitude draws your attention to things that are going right. This can be especially helpful at the start of your day, at the end of your day before you go to sleep, or anytime you are feeling overwhelmed with stress. There are always things to feel good about, if you choose to notice them.

Right now, try to think of three things for which you are grateful today. Say them out loud, write them down on paper or in a journal, or share them with someone else to truly reflect on them. (This could include your health, your family's health, friendships you cherish, a kindness you noticed today, a laugh you shared with someone, or a job well done.)

Creativity

Finally, one effective way to reduce stress in your mind and body is to find a creative outlet for it. This can take many forms, including:

- **Art:** drawing, painting, sculpting, scrapbooking
- **Music:** listening to music, writing/creating music, playing an instrument
- **Writing:** journaling, writing short stories, poems, song or rap lyrics, creating comic books or graphic novels, writing fan fiction
- **Photography:** taking photos, editing photos, sharing or publishing photos
- **Dance:** composing choreography, dancing alone or with others
- **Culinary arts:** cooking or baking
- **Singing:** alone for fun, taking formal lessons, joining a choir
- **Acting:** taking lessons, joining an improv group, participating in theater
- **Design:** fashion design, interior design, architecture

When trying these 10 strategies, do you notice any difference in your body or mind? Do you feel less tense and more relaxed? Is your mind calmer and clearer? With practice, these effects will become stronger and more obvious. Consider adding some (or all) of these strategies to your "backpack" as essential supplies for your journey to a happier, calmer life.

Up Close and Personal with Stress: Identifying Your Stressors

Now that you understand how stress affects your brain and body, let's explore how it affects your thoughts, feelings, and behaviors. These checklists will help identify the stressors in your life and how you've been responding to them. You've probably learned one or two helpful coping strategies along the way, that you can identify in the checklists. You've probably also been using unhelpful strategies that you'd like to replace with more successful techniques, and the checklists help sort those out, too. In case you think of one or two other things that aren't listed, you'll find some space to write them in.

Check off all items that apply to you:

WHAT STRESSES ME OUT?

☐ Thinking of all of the schoolwork I have to keep up with makes me feel like I'll never get through it.

☐ I feel like I can't keep balancing academics, sports, activities, and a social life.

- [ ] I wonder if my parents and teachers are proud of me, and I worry that I'm not living up to their expectations.

- [ ] I feel under constant stress to be perfect, which is exhausting.

- [ ] Having to perform in front of other people (public speaking, sports, acting, music) gives me a paralyzing feeling of stage fright.

- [ ] Trying to figure out my future plans for college and a career stresses me out.

- [ ] While I'd like to have more friends, the thought of meeting new people makes me too nervous to try.

- [ ] I worry that I may never experience a romantic relationship like I see others enjoying.

- [ ] If I'm in an argument with someone, I start stressing myself out thinking that I did something wrong.

- [ ] When I see conflict in my family, I worry that I'm the cause.

- [ ] When I see others living exciting lives, I worry that I'll never have what they have.

- [ ] I feel like I can't always be myself around other people; it's easier to be my "true" self online, by text, or when I'm alone.

- [ ] People tease, make fun of, or bully me, and I worry about the next time it will happen.

- [ ] Sometimes I worry that I'm different from everyone else, as if there's something wrong with me.

- [ ] Sometimes I'm scared that I can't control my impulses to do things I later regret.

- [ ] I'm stressed out about my body and my looks because I'm not happy with what I see in the mirror.

- [ ] It's really hard for me to deal with changes in my life, such as moving, changing schools, or starting a new job.

- [ ] I worry about money, health, safety, or natural disasters.

- [ ] I find myself worrying about my health or the health and safety of my loved ones.

- [ ] Sometimes I have random anxiety attacks for no reason at all, and I worry that another panic attack could happen at any time.

☐ I don't always feel safe in my home, in my neighborhood, at school, or out in the world.

☐ I feel like I've never gotten over a bad thing or things that happened to me; it still bothers me to this day.

☐ _____

☐ _____

Look over the items you checked in this list. Do you see common themes? Write down any themes or patterns you may have noticed in your personal stressors:

_____

_____

_____

_____

HOW I COPE

☐ I distract myself with movies, TV shows, video games, or social media to avoid focusing on what I'm stressed about.

☐ I seek out funny or cute things to make me laugh and break some tension.

☐ I sometimes skip classes or stay home for the day to avoid school stress.

☐ I talk to friends, a sibling, and/or my parents when I can't figure out how to solve a problem.

☐ I try to exercise or go for a walk, run, or bike ride to clear my head of stress.

☐ I practice yoga or stretching to help me relax.

☐ In front of other people, I make jokes or pretend that I'm feeling happier than I really am to seem more appealing.

☐ I drink alcohol, vape, or smoke cigarettes or marijuana to escape from all of my stress for a little while.

☐ I have outbursts of crying, yelling, or physical aggression when too much stress has been bottling up.

☐ I use prayer to help relieve some of the burden I feel.

- [ ] I use creative hobbies like reading, writing stories, making music, taking photos, drawing, or painting to release some of my feelings.

- [ ] I sometimes avoid arguing with family members or friends just so I don't upset anyone or cause problems.

- [ ] I eat my favorite foods to comfort myself.

- [ ] I eat impulsively and sometimes lose control, and then feel guilty about it.

- [ ] I restrict or otherwise change my eating to feel in control.

- [ ] I sleep more than usual or take naps just to avoid feeling so stressed.

- [ ] I try to go outside or to a different place for a change of scenery to clear my head.

- [ ] I withdraw from other people and just spend time alone.

- [ ] I procrastinate on things that cause me stress, such as studying for a test or starting a big project.

- [ ] I take a shower or bath to calm down.

- [ ] I focus on grooming or putting on nice clothes to make myself feel more confident.

- [ ] I use cutting, burning, or other self-harm behaviors to get a sense of relief when I feel overwhelmed.

- [ ] I try to relax by taking deep breaths or meditating.

- [ ] I spend time taking care of, cuddling, or playing with a pet.

- [ ] _____

- [ ] _____

Look over the items you checked in this list. Which strategies are helpful and successful, making you feel calmer and more capable? Could you try to use these more often? Which strategies do you commonly turn to that aren't too healthy? Are you motivated to try something else instead?

_____

_____

_____

_____

IT'S A MARATHON, NOT A SPRINT

Today, you are at the starting line of your own race. The two checklists you just completed were a reflective practice to help you identify where you are, and where you want to be.

First, take a moment to feel proud of the successful coping strategies you already use; the skills you have can help you use coping strategies more mindfully in the future. For instance, plenty of teens are surprised to hear that simple things like taking a shower or a nap are actually highly recommended stress-reducing strategies.

Secondly, note the coping strategies you use that are not so successful. Are you ready to try something new instead?

The marathon ahead is made up of small steps you take on a daily basis. Maybe you try out deep breathing before an exam, or you choose to exercise to blow off steam after an argument with a parent. You have to train every day, and some days will be better than others, but you are always moving forward. Just like an athlete builds up endurance for weeks before a marathon, daily practice will help you achieve your greater goal of feeling less stressed in your life. Persistence pays off.

Imagine your personal finish line: What will your life look like when you are confident that you can handle stress with ease? Maybe you'll enjoy spending time with friends without worrying about their opinions of you; maybe scrolling through social media will create more feelings of pleasure than insecurity; maybe fear won't stop you from asking out your crush; maybe you'll feel a balance between schoolwork, responsibilities, hobbies, and an active social life; maybe you'll feel excitement instead of dread at the top of a competitive game; maybe instead of feeling guilty about procrastinating, you'll feel motivated to work toward goals like studying for a standardized test or applying for college.

The next section will help you envision that personal finish line, one where stress no longer holds you back.

IMAGINE A LIFE WITH LESS STRESS

When you're under stress overload, it's easy to feel lost. Take some time now to find your direction. As we clear the path ahead of you one step at a time, imagine your ultimate destination—your life with less stress and more peace. The following questions can help you paint a mental picture.

In a life with less stress . . .

How will you feel? How will you act? Describe your less-stressed self.

_____

_____

_____

_____

How will you spend your time? What activities will be fun, relaxing, and pleasurable?

_____

_____

_____

_____

What will you do to take care of your health (both physical and emotional) to ensure you're ready to manage stress?

_____

_____

_____

_____

Can you imagine yourself successfully handling conflicts with others? How might you solve interpersonal problems more effectively?

_____

_____

_____

_____

Success Stories: Teens Building Confidence

MICHAEL'S STORY

Michael is trying to enjoy the summer after eighth grade graduation but can't stop worrying about next year. It's never been easy to make friends, and he imagines it'll be even harder as a freshman in a crowded high school. When Michael starts to notice more stomachaches (his body's stress cue), he decides to take charge of his anxiety. First, he chooses a mantra to calm himself: *"Courage is not the absence of fear but moving forward in spite of it."* He starts writing a graphic novel that visualizes a successful freshman year. He's nervous about sharing it but decides to post images on social media. When he receives negative comments, he notices a stomachache coming on and calms himself with deep breathing. Michael also shifts his focus to the positive comments and reaches out to thank each person for their support. This reconnects Michael with friends from elementary school, which helps him feel less lonely. Although he still walks into his first day with some nervousness, remembering his mantra helps him remain confident and steady.

NOELLE'S STORY

Noelle is a self-proclaimed "worrywart" who stresses about how she'll perform on, well, everything. She stays home from parties to avoid conversations with people. She hasn't gotten her learner's permit because she's too afraid of failing her driver's test. Now, Noelle has been offered a great part-time job related to her passion—photography—but she's worried she'll somehow mess it up. After talking with her mom, Noelle realizes that she doesn't want her nervousness to hold her back from enjoying life, and she decides to confront her fears. To calm her body and quiet her mind, Noelle watches online videos guiding her through autogenic relaxation while she focuses on the words "I am calm." Noelle also decides to practice daily gratitude by writing down one thing she's grateful for (like the photography job) and showing gratitude toward one person (like thanking her mom for driving lessons). With these changes, Noelle gradually feels more confident facing uncomfortable situations that she knows can bring her happiness.

Success Stories: Teens Building Confidence

TAYLOR'S STORY

Taylor is a college freshman and away from home for the first time. Taylor always got good grades in school, despite lots of procrastination and cramming. After the first month of college, as the excitement wore off and the workload picked up, Taylor became overwhelmed. It grew harder to focus on studying and to resist the temptation to hang out in the student lounge or sleep through an early morning lecture. After failing midterms, Taylor was in "stress overload" and decided to focus on school and self-care. First, Taylor started going to the campus gym to swim, run, or lift weights. Next, Taylor met with an academic adviser to create a week-by-week plan for the rest of the semester, so catching up didn't feel too overwhelming. Taylor started to use a guided-imagery app at night to fall asleep, making it easier to wake up in time for morning lectures. By the end of the semester, Taylor felt back on track and more confident about handling the stress of semesters to come.

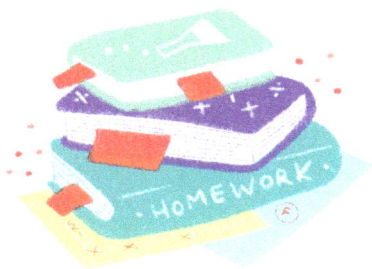

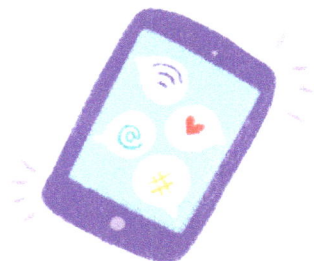

Can you visualize yourself feeling confident and excited when facing challenging times, such as preparing for a big test, handling responsibilities at work, or performing in front of others? How might you use anxiety as a driving force?

_____

_____

_____

_____

When stressful thoughts arise around things you can't control, such as how the future plays out, how might you stay calm and in control of anxious feelings?

_____

_____

_____

_____

For a moment, try to hold on to this visual image of your life with less stress and more peace. Hold on to the sense of calm it may bring you, or the energizing motivation that may arise from that new sense of hopefulness.

Along your journey, when you need a boost of encouragement, enthusiasm, or inspiration, read over your answers to this exercise to call to mind this positive mindset, which can motivate you to keep moving forward.

You may also reread your answers after you've reached the end of this workbook to reflect on all the progress you've made in your journey.

TODAY IS TRAINING DAY #1

Now that you've created an image of your life with less stress, let's make today the first day of creating that reality. Keeping in mind the 10 stress-reducing strategies we've already discussed, think about small changes you can make to your daily life. What can you do to reduce stress and feel better today? Right now?

This will likely involve doing some things in a different way than you're used to, or even in the opposite way. Here are some examples:

If you usually . . .	Then try . . .
distract your attention away from stressful things (for example, procrastinating on schoolwork by scrolling through social media)	breaking down the overwhelming task into smaller, more manageable steps to get it done, like studying for 20 minutes tonight

If you usually . . .	Then try . . .
avoid an anxiety-provoking activity or event (such as skipping a party for fear of socializing)	showing up, if only for a few minutes, to prove to yourself that it's not so bad (or maybe even a great time!)

If you usually . . .	Then try . . .
withdraw, keeping your feelings to yourself	reaching out to a friend or family member, even if just to say something like, "I'm feeling really stressed right now." You might be surprised by how good it feels to connect with someone in hard times.

Much like the 10 techniques we discussed, I encourage you to try a new strategy at least once or twice to see if it's helpful. Remember that you need practice to start benefiting from these new skills you're learning.

CONCLUSION

Congratulations! You've learned all about how the basic stress response affects your brain and body, and started to pay closer attention to how you personally experience stress. You have gained knowledge about techniques that are proven to reduce stress, and you've put some thought into how you might use these new skills in your daily life. Part 2 will guide you through exercises that help you practice your new skills in a way that works for you.

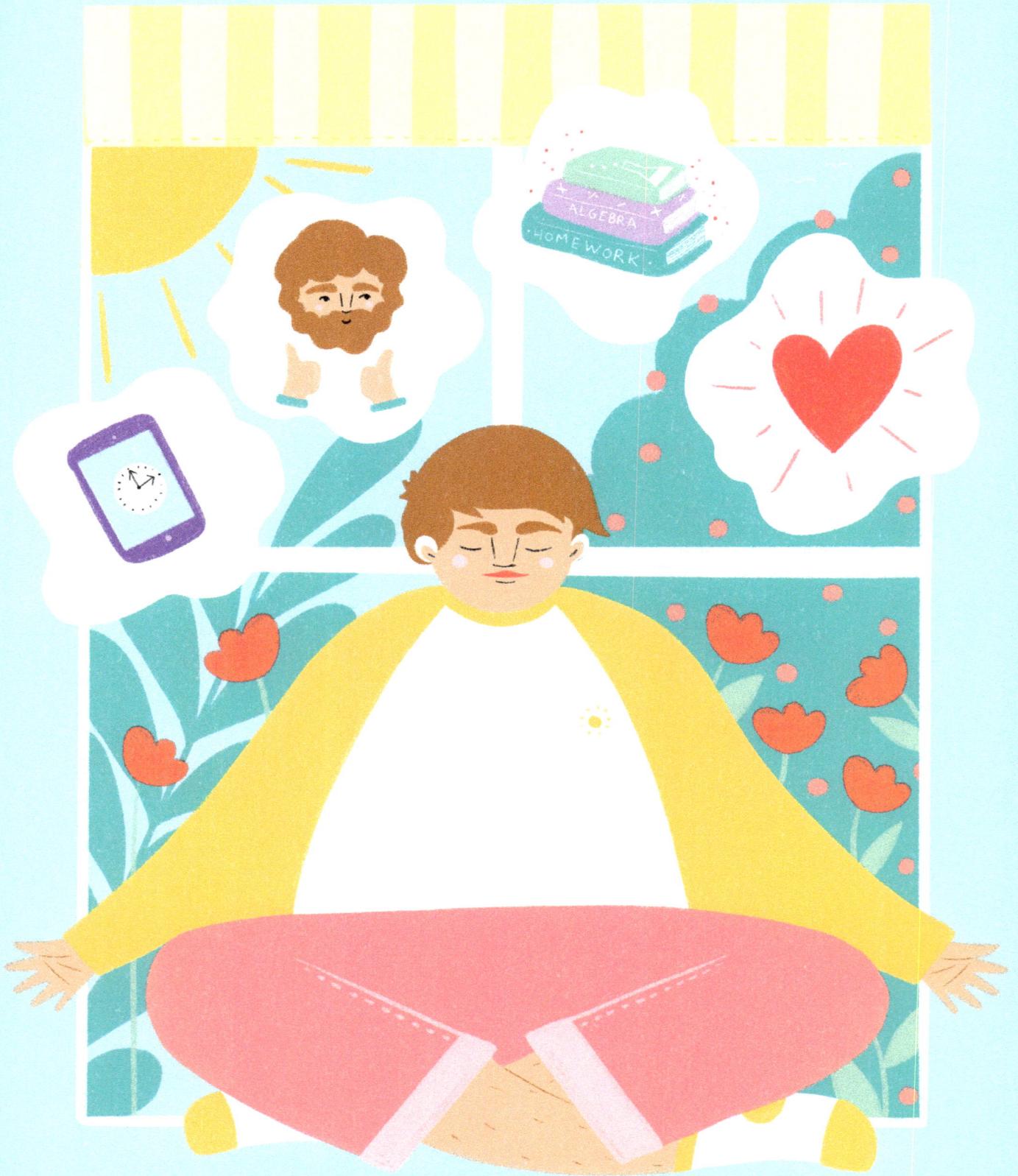

PART 2

Managing Stress on Your Journey to a More Peaceful Life

Now that you understand how stress personally affects you, let's practice new and different ways of responding. Part 2 will focus on themes like self-care, managing emotions, discovering personal values you want to live by, communication and problem-solving, conquering negative thinking, and maintaining healthy relationships.

Remember to be patient with yourself. These are long-term life skills that take time to develop. But each day is a new opportunity to take care of yourself by managing stress.

continued ▶

ACTIVITY 1:

Daily Self-Care and Balancing Parts of the Whole

Self-care as a whole is made up of many different parts, but they are all interconnected. The following tool, known as a self-care wheel, illustrates six different categories including: mental health, physical health, creativity/spirituality, relationships, environment, and personal growth. By caring for each part, the whole person stays in balance. In the white space next to each category, fill in one idea you can start practicing today.

As you complete more activities throughout this workbook, you'll discover new self-care techniques to add within each category. In the end, we'll revisit this self-care wheel, which will become more balanced with time and practice.

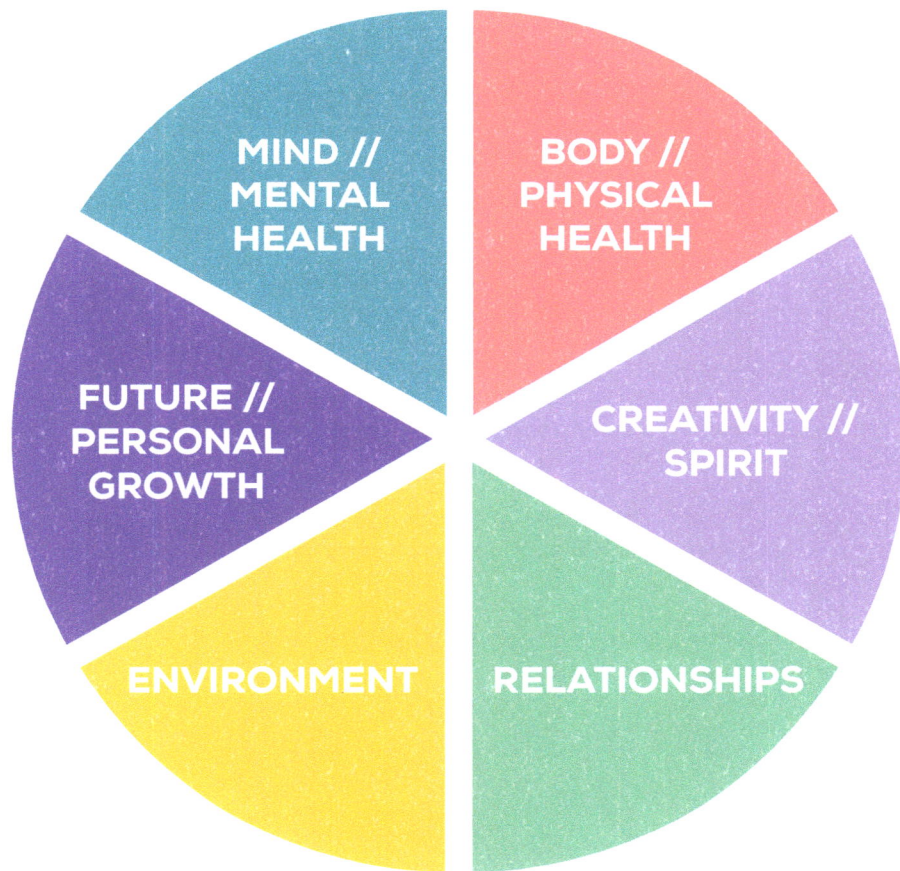

ACTIVITY 2: Self-Care in Times of Stress

While it's important to practice daily self-care, it's absolutely vital to take good care of yourself when you're in stress overload. Take this quiz to see how you take care of yourself when it's most important.

Think of a recent time you were in stress overload. Read each item and circle "true" or "false" for each question:

1.	I made attempts to get enough sleep to stay well-rested.	True	False
2.	I tried my best to eat meals to keep my body healthy.	True	False
3.	I still made time for physical activity, movement, or exercise, even if only for a few minutes.	True	False
4.	I made efforts to take care of my basic hygiene and grooming (showering, combing my hair, wearing clothes I felt good in).	True	False
5.	I made efforts to take care of my environment (keeping my room clean, doing laundry, cleaning up dishes after eating).	True	False
6.	I tried to stick to my daily routine, like showing up to school or my job, even when I didn't feel up to it.	True	False
7.	I made sure to include fun, relaxing, or soothing activities every day, if only for a few minutes, to help me recharge.	True	False
8.	I stayed away from coping mechanisms that I've learned create more problems in the long run for me. (Examples might include drinking alcohol, making impulsive decisions, or behaving aggressively toward others.)	True	False
9.	I reached out to someone such as a friend, family member, therapist, teacher, or coach to let them know I was having a tough time and needed support.	True	False
10.	I was able to set limits with others or stood up for myself in order to keep myself safe and happy.	True	False

Now, count how many "true" responses you circled:

7 to 10 = You are putting in great effort to take care of yourself even when it's most difficult. Keep up the good work!

4 to 6 = You are able to do some healthy and helpful things for yourself when you're under stress. It can be hard for you to keep up self-care when you are overwhelmed. Look closely at your "false" responses. Are you willing to try one or two of these strategies in the future?

0 to 3 = It's hard to care for yourself when you are overwhelmed with stress. It may feel like you don't have the energy, motivation, or ability to overcome daily challenges. Start small: look over your "false" responses and see if there is one new thing you can try out the next time you are in stress overload.

What are some ways you might add more self-care into your daily routines?

_____

_____

_____

_____

_____

_____

_____

_____

ACTIVITY 3: Self-Care Is Sleep

Sleep fuels both your brain and body, but most teens don't get nearly enough (8 to 10 hours is best). Try to calculate your average amount of sleep—is it at least eight hours?

Here are five basic strategies to help you get a good night's sleep, which can boost your mood, increase your energy level, improve your concentration, and help you solve problems more easily. If you implement most of these habits, you'll likely notice positive effects within a day or two. Check off whether you already do each one or if you are interested in starting it:

Sleep Strategy	I already do this!	I'm interested in starting this.
Keep a routine. Even on weekends, try to fall asleep at the same time at night and wake up around the same time in the morning.		
Avoid daytime naps. Try your best not to nap, but if you must, stick to a 20-minute "power nap" before 5 p.m.		
Use your bed only for sleep. Try to use your bed only for sleeping and not for doing homework, playing video games, or any other alert activity.		
Relax before bedtime. Have a light snack without sugar or caffeine, avoid screens, and engage in a soothing activity like taking a shower, listening to an audiobook, or practicing deep breathing and mindfulness.		
Create a sleep haven. Keep your room dark, cool, and quiet for the best-quality sleep. Try listening to a soothing sound, such as a fan, calm music, nature sounds, or a podcast specifically designed to help people sleep.		

How else might you make sleep a priority and part of your self-care routine?

_____

_____

_____

_____

_____

_____

_____

_____

_____

_____

ACTIVITY 4: Self-Care Is Eating to Fuel Your Day

Healthy eating—including what, when, and how much you eat—has a huge effect on both your brain and body. Especially during times of high stress, it's important to make small efforts throughout the day to fuel our brains and bodies with food that helps us take on everything we want and need to do.

Here's a sample daily plan for eating to help structure your day and combat hunger-related stress.

- 7:30 a.m. **Breakfast.** *I'll make sure to eat breakfast, even if it's just a few bites (yogurt with fruit and nuts, granola bar with a glass of milk, fruit smoothie with spinach).*

- 9:00 a.m. **Hydrate.** *I'll flavor my water with some orange slices and ice and fill up my bottle so I can carry water around with me all day.*

- 12:30 p.m. **Balanced Lunch.** *I'll try to eat a full meal, instead of snacking, to help with focus and energy for the rest of the afternoon. I'll add protein (turkey, chicken, beans) with complex carbohydrates (veggies, fruit, whole wheat bread or crackers).*

- 3:30 p.m. **Healthy Snack.** *Instead of reaching for salty or sweet snacks after school, I'll choose a healthier snack (carrots and hummus, apple slices and peanut butter, popcorn and a smoothie).*

- 6:00 p.m. **Balanced Dinner.** *I'll eat a full meal, with protein, veggies, and complex carbs so that I'm not overly hungry for snacks later on.*

- 9:00 p.m. **Light Snack.** *I'll try to eat a lighter, healthier snack in the evening that will help me sleep (milk, cheese, whole grain toast with a little jam, nuts).*

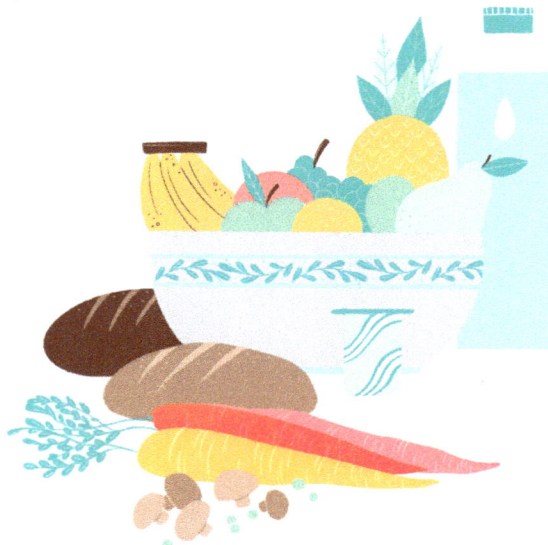

Use the blank lines to create your own plan with ideas you already use or would like to try.

_____

_____

_____

_____

_____

_____

_____

_____

_____

_____

_____

_____

_____

_____

_____

_____

_____

_____

_____

_____

ACTIVITY 5: Self-Care Is Movement

Physical activity is a proven stress reliever that benefits both your body and mind. You might find it easier to add physical activity to your life if it feels more like fun than work. Adding a partner can be especially helpful for motivating you to keep at it!

Check out this sample daily physical activity calendar.

Sun	Mon	Tues	Wed	Thurs	Fri	Sat
	1 Take a walk with a friend after school	2	3 Ride my bike	4	5 "Yoga Friday" (20 mins.)	6
7 Go for a jog with Dad	8	9 Play pickup basketball at the park	10	11	12 "Yoga Friday" (20 mins.)	13 25 mins. on the treadmill
14	15 Dance to my party playlist (30 mins.)	16	17 Skateboard	18	19 "Yoga Friday" (20 mins.)	20
21 Open swim at community center	22	23 Push-ups, lunges, squats (30 mins.)	24	25 Ride my scooter	26 "Yoga Friday" (20 mins.)	27
28 Hike the local park trails with a friend	29	30 Ride bikes with my sister				

Use the blank chart to create your own calendar with ideas you already use or would like to try.

Sun	Mon	Tues	Wed	Thurs	Fri	Sat
	1	2	3	4	5	6
7	8	9	10	11	12	13
14	15	16	17	18	19	20
21	22	23	24	25	26	27
28	29	30				

ACTIVITY 6: Tuning In to Your Stress Cues

When you pay attention to self-care on a daily basis, it becomes easier to recognize your stress levels. And being able to identify the situations that cause you stress is an important first step in learning how to better cope in the future. For instance, you may learn to prevent some stressful situations altogether by asking a friend or parent for support, or by using techniques like deep breathing to keep yourself calm and confident. Take a moment to review the following common stress cues and check the ones that apply to you. If you think of others, write those down, too.

SITUATIONS THAT OFTEN TRIGGER STRESS:

☐   Social gatherings

☐   Performing in front of others

☐   Schoolwork

☐   My job

☐   Feeling too busy/not having enough time

☐   Arguing with friends or family

☐   Relationship trouble

☐   Uncertainty about my future

☐   Feeling unhappy with my body or looks

☐   _____

BODY CUES THAT SIGNAL STRESS:

☐   My heart races.

☐   I feel hot and sweaty.

☐   I tremble.

☐   My breathing is faster and shallower.

☐   My muscles tense up.

☐   I fidget or feel restless (bounce leg, tap fingers, bite fingernails, pace, etc.).

☐   _____

THOUGHT CUES THAT SIGNAL STRESS:

- ☐ My mind races with thoughts that I can't slow down.

- ☐ It's hard to focus or concentrate.

- ☐ I feel constantly worried.

- ☐ I become forgetful and disorganized.

- ☐ I make impulsive decisions without thinking first.

- ☐ I become pessimistic and fear the worst outcome.

- ☐ _____

BEHAVIOR CUES THAT SIGNAL STRESS:

- ☐ I withdraw from other people.

- ☐ I notice changes in my eating.

- ☐ I notice changes in my sleep.

- ☐ I procrastinate or avoid stress-provoking things.

- ☐ I become moody, irritable, or easily annoyed.

- ☐ I cry more often than usual or at things that I normally wouldn't.

- ☐ _____

What other ways do you tune in to your stress cues?

_____

_____

_____

_____

_____

_____

ACTIVITY 7: Reading Your Stress Thermometer

Now that you've learned more about your personal stress cues, the next step is to notice their intensity. Observing how much stress affects your thoughts, body, or behaviors can help you determine just how close you are to reaching stress overload. Imagine if you had a thermometer that could measure your level of stress in different situations.

10. _____

_____

_____

_____

6. Argued with Mom about
   college applications

5. _____

_____

_____

_____

1. _____

10. _____

_____

_____

_____

6. Tense muscles, felt hot, I
   raised my voice and cursed

5. _____

_____

_____

_____

1. _____

A small stressor, like being called on in class, can cause a quick rush of body heat that dissipates quickly (maybe 2 on a scale of 1 to 10). On the other hand, the first few weeks after a breakup can cause constant worry, sadness, moodiness, and poor eating and sleeping habits (maybe 8 on the scale).

On the left side of the thermometer, fill in the blanks with examples of recent stressors that hit 1, 5, and 10. On the right side of the thermometer, fill in the stress cues you noticed in that situation.

ACTIVITY 8: Lowering Your Stress Temperature

Once you become more familiar with your stress levels (what a 2 feels like as compared to a 9), the next step is to learn to use coping skills to prevent your stress from rising too high. As soon as you notice your stress temperature rising, immediately try a relaxation strategy (see examples on pages 9–14) to stay cool and in control.

Identify which of the following coping strategies can help you at each level of stress on the thermometer. If you have ideas for how these strategies might be useful in certain situations, write them below.

- Deep breathing
- Five-senses mindfulness
- Visualization exercise
- Movement/physical activity

- Progressive muscle relaxation (PMR)
- Repeating your mantra
- Practice a gratitude exercise
- Use a creative outlet

_____

_____

_____

_____

_____

_____

_____

_____

_____

_____

ACTIVITY 9:

Accepting Anger (and the Emotions Behind It)

In therapy, we often use a visual image of the tip of an iceberg to describe the fact that anger is a "surface emotion." That means we can be quick to feel mad, but if we slow down to think about it, there's likely much more going on below the surface. Take a look at this example of an anger iceberg, showing a variety of feelings that might underlie the anger:

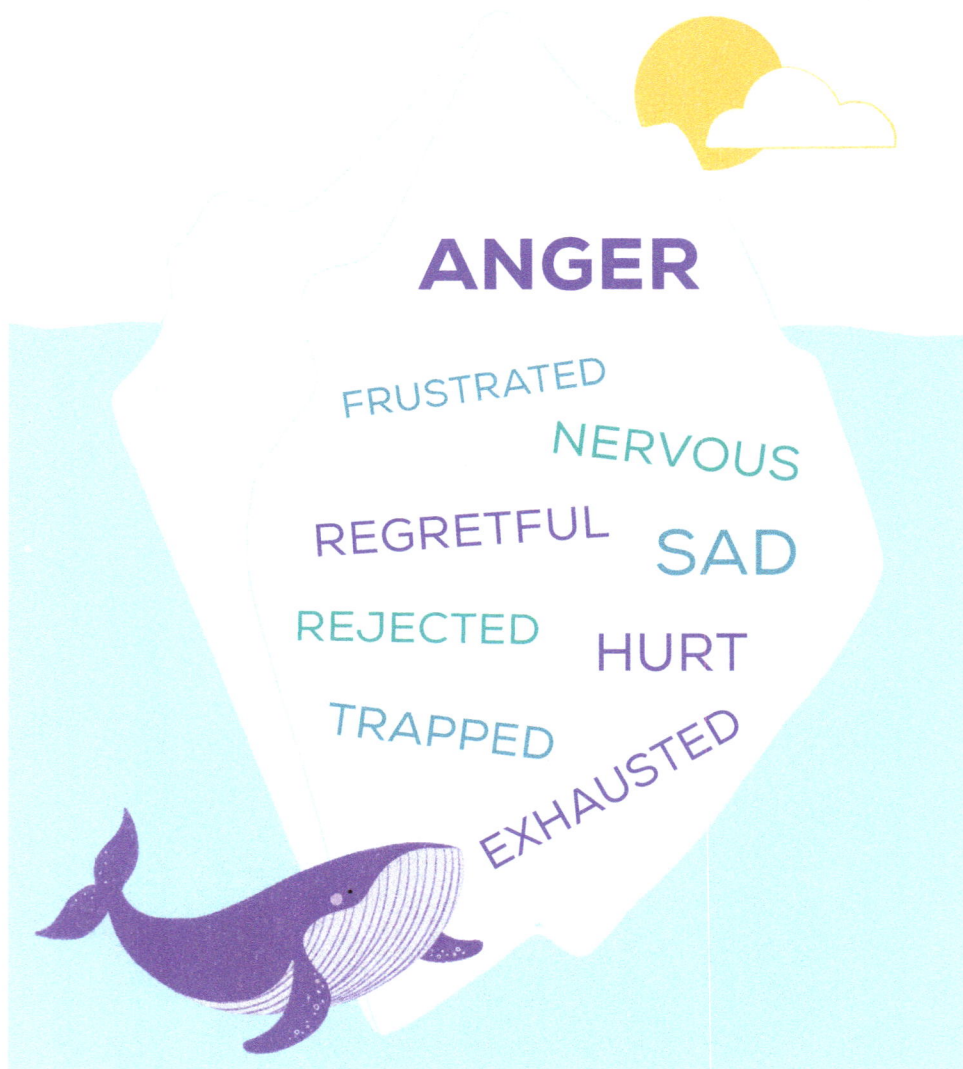

ANGER

FRUSTRATED
NERVOUS
REGRETFUL
SAD
REJECTED
HURT
TRAPPED
EXHAUSTED

Read the example, then complete the activity with one of your own experiences.

Kai wasn't feeling well and skipped her friend's party one Friday night. While scrolling Instagram, a picture suddenly popped up of Kai's girlfriend at the party kissing someone else on the cheek. A rush of anger swept over Kai, who immediately sent a chain of furious texts about wanting to break up. After a few minutes, Kai started to regret that decision, realizing it was an impulsive jump to conclusions. Kai filled out the anger iceberg worksheet from therapy to figure out what feelings were truly behind the anger.

Think of a recent time when you felt very angry, maybe an 8, 9, or 10 on your anger scale. Try the iceberg activity to see if you can identify deeper feelings that contributed to the anger:

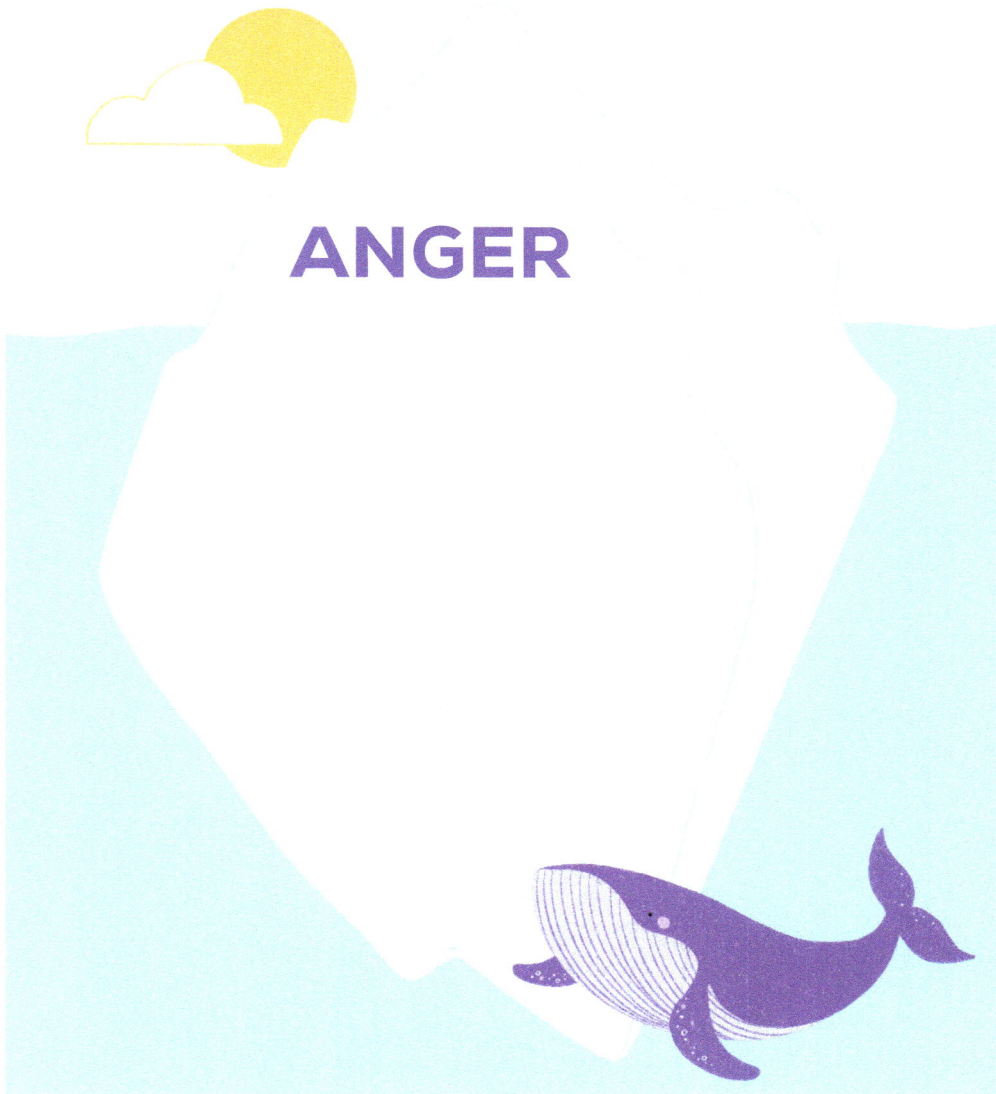

ANGER

ACTIVITY 10: Name That Emotion

Beyond recognizing stress, you can also use the visual image of a thermometer to measure a variety of emotions. When your stress thermometer rises, it can be very helpful to explore if any other strong feelings are contributing to your stress. Consider the following feelings:

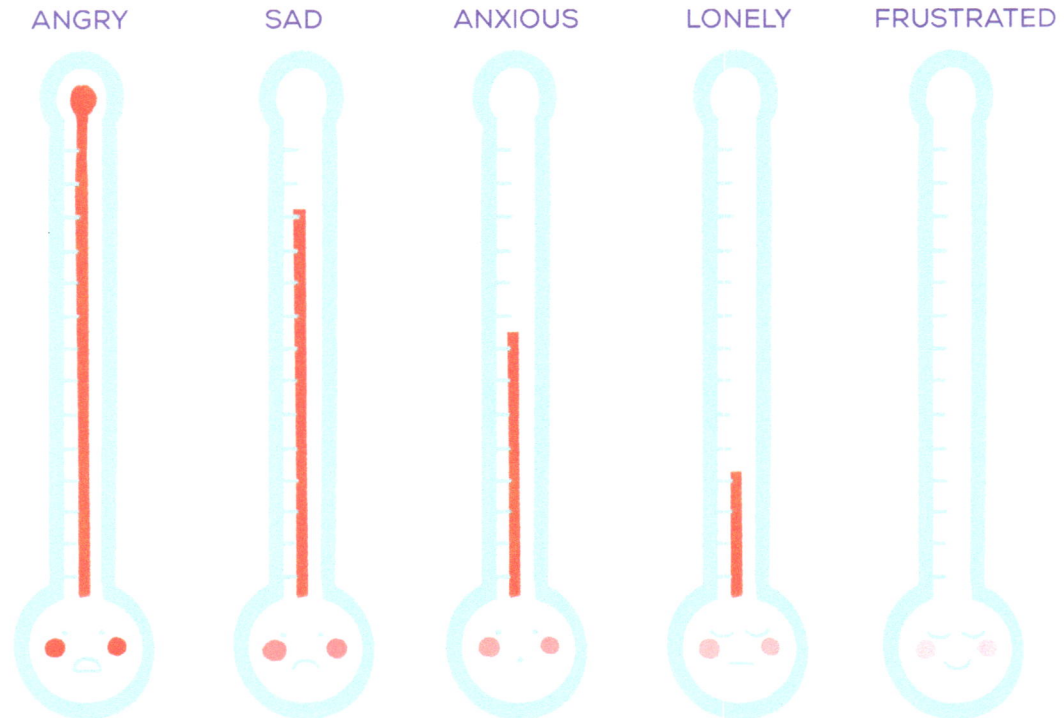

ANGRY   SAD   ANXIOUS   LONELY   FRUSTRATED

Now look back at activity 7: Reading Your Stress Thermometer (page 38), where you filled in situations that caused a 1, 5, and 10 on your stress scale. Were other emotions involved? If so, name the emotion(s) and rate how intense they were on the emotional thermometer.

_____

_____

_____

_____

_____

ACTIVITY 11: Staying Active against Depression

Let's take a moment to talk about depression, specifically how it can affect teens. Many people, including adults, tend to think that depression "looks like" crying a lot, sleeping all day, and living every day in a "black hole." This is not always an accurate picture, and it's certainly not always true for teens.

Symptoms of depression in teenagers tend to include:

- Frequent physical aches and pains (headaches, stomach-aches, muscle aches)

- Feeling agitated and restless, like you can't relax

- Loss of pleasure, especially in things you used to enjoy

- Changes to sleep habits (sleeping much more or much less than usual)

- Changes to appetite or eating habits

- Constant low energy and feeling tired or run-down

- Trouble concentrating, feeling distracted

- Irritability, moodiness, being quick to anger

- Withdrawing from friends and family

- Lack of motivation to get started on anything

- Feeling guilty

- Feeling empty

While all of the techniques in this workbook can help relieve mild depression, the most effective strategy is to "get active" in two specific ways.

1. **Get socially active.** Fight back against the urge to isolate, and instead surround yourself with other people. This can mean talking about your feelings with a trusted adult, hanging out with a friend, or simply being in the same room with your family members. List three people you can spend time with when you're feeling down:

_____

_____

_____

continued ▶

2. **Get behaviorally active.** Push yourself to get up and going on some activity, even if you aren't feeling motivated. This could be showering and getting dressed, cleaning your room, reaching out to a friend, going for a walk, or engaging in a favorite hobby. Once you've started the action, you may notice your motivation follows. List three activities that could help you feel more energized:

_____

_____

_____

IMPORTANT NOTE: *If you ever find it too difficult to help yourself out of a depressed mood, if you are feeling hopeless, if you are harming yourself in any way, or if you have thoughts about suicide, it's important to share this information with a parent, teacher, therapist, doctor, or trusted adult right away. Skip ahead to the Crisis Resources section (page 123) now to find options for immediate support.*

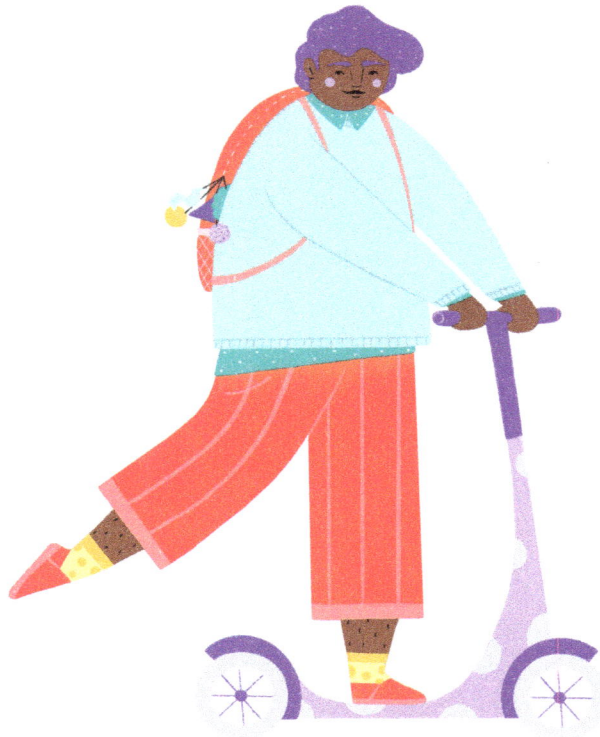

Creating Calm through Soothing Sensations

When you feel overwhelmed with general stress along with deeper, more negative feelings like anger, fear, sadness, or loneliness, one immediate self-soothing strategy is to use your five senses to calm your mind and your body. You can use this strategy in any stressful situation to immediately relieve stress by exerting control over your attention. Let go of worry about the future or regrets about the past by purely focusing on the present moment. Prepare for the next time you need to soothe your senses by identifying the things you'll use:

1. **Vision.** What is soothing to look at? (For example: a favorite picture; nature, flowers, a tree, or the sky; a piece of artwork; a funny video)

_____

_____

_____

_____

_____

2. **Hearing.** What is soothing to listen to? (For example: music, nature sounds like waves or raindrops, a clock ticking, a friend's voice, a video of cute animal sounds)

_____

_____

_____

_____

_____

continued ▶

3. **Touch.** What is soothing to touch or feel? (For example: warm water in a shower or bath, lotion, an animal, a comfy bed or couch, or a stress ball or other fidget-friendly object)

_____

_____

_____

_____

_____

4. **Smell.** What is soothing to smell? (For example: a candle, scented lotion, your favorite food cooking, flowers, or other things outside)

_____

_____

_____

_____

_____

5. **Taste.** What is soothing to taste? (For example: your favorite meal, a gum or mint, tea or hot chocolate)

_____

_____

_____

_____

_____

ACTIVITY 13: Creative Keys to Help Process Your Feelings

When you're overwhelmed with stress on top of deeper, more negative feelings (like anger, fear, sadness, or loneliness), another helpful coping strategy is to express yourself creatively. This helps you identify your emotions, process how you think and feel, gain some control, and relieve some tension by channeling your energy elsewhere. There are countless ways to use your feelings as fuel for creativity.

And don't be afraid to try new things. It can feel awkward at first but may become very rewarding in the end. Put a checkmark next to each idea to indicate which creative outlets you already engage in, which you're interested in trying, and which you're not:

Creative Outlet	Yes, I already do this.	I would like to try this.	No, I'm not interested.
Art: drawing, painting, sculpting, scrapbooking			
Music: listening to, creating, or playing music; singing, taking singing lessons, or joining a choir			
Writing: writing journal entries, short stories, poems, song or rap lyrics, comic books or graphic novels, or fan fiction			
Photography: taking, editing, sharing, and publishing photos			
Dance: composing choreography, dancing alone or with others			
Culinary arts: cooking or baking, devising new recipes			
Acting: taking lessons, joining an improv group, participating in theater			
Design: designing and/or making clothes, jewelry, or interior decor			

continued ▶

Now, think about how you can actively start to try one (or more) of these new creative pursuits. Can you look up them up online? Talk to a family member or teacher about them? Write down some ways you can begin actively exploring new ways to channel your stress and get creative in the process.

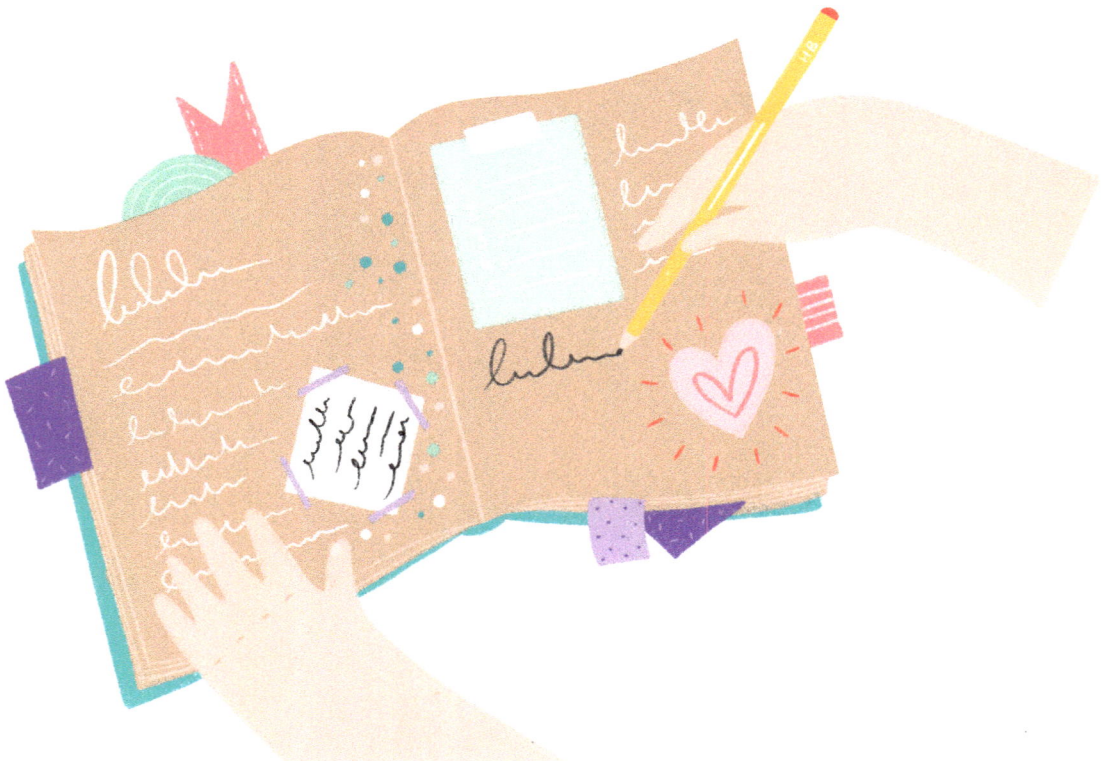

_____

_____

_____

_____

_____

_____

_____

_____

ACTIVITY 14: Share the Burden

One final coping strategy to manage deeper, more negative feelings that contribute to stress is to reach out to your social support network. You can choose to describe as little or as much as you feel comfortable with, from just saying, "I'm feeling pretty stressed out, can we just chill?" to going into full detail about your feelings. Here's a framework for helping you figure out what you need: the five Ws of seeking support.

1. **When** do you need help? How will you know it's time to reach out, before you reach stress overload?

_____

_____

_____

_____

2. **Why** do you need help right now? Think through what exactly is stressing you out at the moment. What problems are on your mind?

_____

_____

_____

_____

3. **What** kind of help do you need? Someone to distract you, make you laugh, listen, understand your situation, help brainstorm ideas, give you advice?

_____

_____

_____

_____

continued ▶

4. **Who** can provide you with support—parents, siblings, friends, a romantic partner, teacher, coach, community leader, religious leader, therapist, doctor?

_____

_____

_____

_____

5. **Where** can you receive help? Through a phone call, texting, face-to-face visit? At home, school, community center, place of worship?

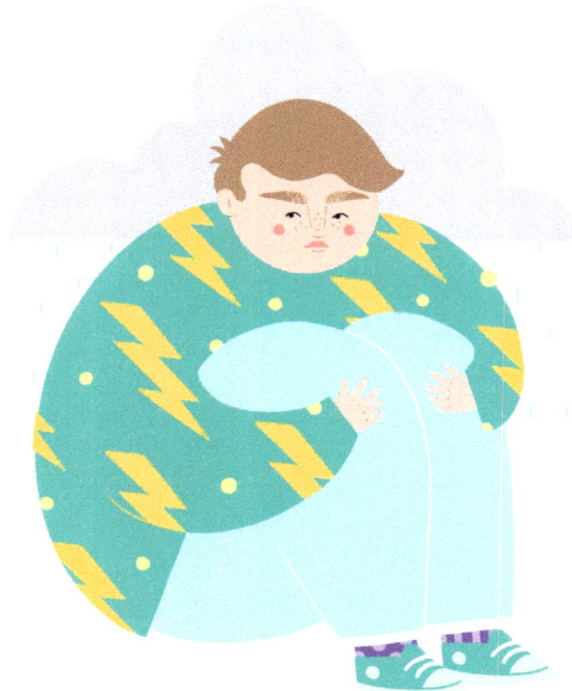

_____

_____

_____

_____

ACTIVITY 15:

Acknowledging the Difference between Facts and Feelings

There are some stressful situations that we simply can't change, no matter how hard we try. For instance, think of your least favorite teacher of all time—did you feel stuck in a difficult school year? If you can't change the situation, figuring out a way to manage it is the next best thing. Acceptance and commitment therapy (ACT) encourages us to manage the stressors in our lives by following the ACT formula: accept your thoughts, feelings, and reactions; commit to your values; take action.

ACT encourages you to fully accept the thoughts and feelings that arise in your mind instead of avoiding them. This can be an especially empowering strategy when you find yourself in a stressful situation beyond your control. Realizing that a feeling is *just a feeling, not a fact*, can help take away its power.

For example, after submitting college applications, you might experience high stress levels since the "waiting game" can be hard to tolerate. The truth is, potential worst-case scenarios are *just worries, not facts.* Instead of obsessing, doubting, and overthinking, it can be freeing to accept that you've done all you can and to let go of the anxiety.

In the following table, think of one or two situations that are out of your control. Write down a thought that helps you fully accept the situation and release your negative feelings.

Situation Beyond My Control	Thoughts That Help Me Accept and Let Go
I want to ask my crush out on a date, but I'm not sure if they like me, and they might say no.	If they say no, it will be hurtful, but I'll be okay.

ACTIVITY 16: Defining Your Values

ACT also focuses on defining your own personal values: the things in life that you feel are most important, like family relationships, education, creative projects, helping others, or spirituality. Exploring your values can help you choose life directions, and that's what this exercise will help you do. Keep in mind, there's no one set of "correct" values; each person has a unique sense of what is most meaningful.

Read over each item, and write out how important each value is to you at this point in your life. For other areas that might not be covered, fill in the blank examples if you need to.

1. **Family Relationships.** Are you satisfied with your role in family relationships right now? If not, how might you improve this area of your life?

    _____

    _____

    _____

2. **Friendships.** Are you satisfied with the friendships in your life right now? If not, how might you improve this area of your life?

    _____

    _____

    _____

3. **Romantic Relationships.** Are you satisfied with the status of romantic relationships in your life right now? If not, how might you improve this area of your life?

    _____

    _____

    _____

4. **Education.** Are you satisfied with your educational pursuits right now? If not, how might you improve this area of your life?

_____

_____

_____

5. **Recreation/Hobbies/Interests.** Are you satisfied with your current recreational activities right now? If not, how might you improve this area of your life?

_____

_____

_____

6. **Spirituality/Religion/Faith.** Are you satisfied with the status of your spirituality/religion/faith right now? If not, how might you improve this area of your life?

_____

_____

_____

7. **Physical and Mental Health.** Are you satisfied with your physical health and emotional well-being right now? If not, how might you improve this area of your life?

_____

_____

_____

continued ▸

8. **Community/Citizenship.** Are you satisfied with your status as a community/ global citizen right now? If not, how might you improve this area of your life?

_____

_____

_____

9. _____. Are you satisfied with this area of your life? If not, how might you improve it?

_____

_____

_____

10. _____. Are you satisfied with this area of your life? If not, how might you improve it?

_____

_____

_____

ACTIVITY 17: Committing to Take Action

Finally, ACT encourages you to take part in small everyday actions that help you move in a direction that fulfills your values.

Review activity 16: Defining Your Values (page 52) and think about the following questions.

What three values are most important to you? What actions can you commit to today, tomorrow, and this week to get you closer in line with your top three values?

Sample Top Value #1 is friendship.
Actions I can take include:

- *texting a friend I haven't spoken to in a while to see how she's doing*

- *offering help to my classmate who I know has been struggling with schoolwork*

- *starting a conversation with a coworker who seems friendly*

Top Value #1 is _____
Actions I can take include:

_____

_____

_____

Top Value #2 is _____
Actions I can take include:

_____

_____

_____

Top Value #3 is _____
Actions I can take include:

_____

_____

_____

ACTIVITY 18: What's My Communication Style?

You may be familiar with the word "assertiveness" to describe communicating your needs in a healthy way. Assertiveness is a life skill that can help you in many situations, whether it's compromising with your parents, being honest in a romantic relationship, or standing up for yourself with a teacher or a boss. While it might sound a bit daunting to be honest and direct with others, people with assertive communication styles actually report having fewer conflicts in their lives—which translates to less stress.

But assertiveness doesn't have to come naturally; it's a skill that can be learned. It's a happy medium between being passive and being aggressive. Take the following quiz to determine your communication style by reading each item and circling option A, B, or C.

	A	B	C
1. If my friends all agree on an opinion that I disagree with, I would probably:	Be too afraid to speak up for myself and just go along with the group	Speak openly and honestly	Have no problem telling them exactly why I'm right and they're wrong
2. When I try to explain myself to someone in charge, like clearing up a misunderstanding with a teacher that affects my grade, I:	Speak quietly or mumble	Address them confidently	Speak loudly or in a threatening tone
3. When I feel like someone is treating me unfairly and they don't understand my view, I:	Find it hard to explain myself or completely avoid the conversation	Can disagree respectfully and calmly	Might interrupt, shout, or use aggressive language or actions
4. When I am meeting a new person, especially in an unfamiliar crowd like a party, I:	Find it hard to maintain eye contact and/or express myself at all	Can easily maintain eye contact and/or express myself freely	Express myself forcefully; make strong eye contact or stare them down so they know I'm not intimidated

		A	B	C
5.	When others ask me for my opinion, even on something simple like what to eat, I tend to:	Say "It doesn't matter to me" and defer to whatever they want	Express my opinion, listen to others' opinions, and compromise on a final decision	Insist the final decision is what I want
6.	If I notice that a friend always wants to talk about their own problems and never really listens to me, I:	Don't mind so much; their needs are probably more important than mine	Express that I'd like more balance in the friendship, because both of our needs are important	Would stop talking to them entirely because my needs are the most important

If you circled mostly A responses: Your style is **passive**. You tend to hold back your own thoughts, opinions, or feelings. You may believe your needs aren't as important as others' or worry about others disliking you for speaking your mind. Try to catch yourself when you're saying, "I don't know" or "It doesn't matter" and practice giving your opinion, which is just as valid as everyone else's!

If you circled mostly B responses: Your style is **assertive**. You strike a nice balance between feeling confident and accepting of other's opinions and needs. This makes it easy for you to compromise, which fulfills everyone's needs.

If you circled mostly C responses: Your style is **aggressive**. You tend to address others forcefully, without considering their feelings. This may help you get your way, but at the cost of losing people who tire of not being heard. Practice listening to others' ideas and trying to see their point of view.

ACTIVITY 19: Defining Your Needs

Living with unmet needs can lead to stress, frustration, anger, and resentment. Becoming more self-aware of your own needs is hugely important to managing stress in your daily life and relationships. A next step is to learn new communication techniques that help you assert your needs in a way that leads to problem-solving (and thus, less stress). The following activities focus on your ability to define your needs, assert yourself, communicate your needs to others, consider others' needs, and collaborate or compromise with others to come to a successful solution.

Here's an example of a potential conflict regarding needs: Adolescence can be a difficult phase when you've outgrown childhood. You might be craving more autonomy (the ability to make your own choices), but you might not feel quite ready to be an independent adult. This can fuel a lot of arguments between teens and parents or family members.

The following statements are common examples of teens wishing they had more control. Place a checkmark next to any that apply to you, and add any other examples you can think of:

☐ I would like to decide how to spend my own time, especially on the weekends.

☐ I can take care of my own things, like keeping my room how I like it.

☐ I would like to make my own choices about my eating habits.

☐ I would like to make my own decisions about my sleeping habits.

☐ I can stay on top of my grades without my parents' over-involvement.

☐ I would like time to myself, when I can count on privacy.

☐ I would like to have my own money and decide how to spend it.

☐ I would like to learn to drive by myself or have the freedom to do so.

☐ _____

☐ _____

☐ _____

Place a star next to the statement that is most important to you right now (we'll come back to it later). The next step, naturally, is getting your needs met, which involves communicating effectively with others. To do that well, it helps to know your communication style.

ACTIVITY 20: Getting Your Needs Met

Learning to be more assertive is a great strategy to enhance your communication with everyone in your life—parents, siblings, friends, romantic partners, teachers, bosses, coaches, and so on. This builds stronger, more supportive relationships that cause less stress and can serve as a source of support in dealing with other stress when it pops up in your life.

Here are five techniques that can help enhance every conversation you have, especially if you are trying to assert your own thoughts, feelings, or needs.

Look back at activity 19: Defining Your Needs (page 58), where you placed a star next to the most important need you'd like to assert right now. Think through how you might use these five techniques to have a productive conversation about your most important need.

1. **Collect your thoughts.** What message are you trying to send to the other person? What is important for them to know?

   Example: I'd like my parents to stop checking my grades through the parent portal so often, then reminding me of assignments that are due. I want them to know that I can handle it myself, and that it makes me feel like they don't trust me, or that they don't believe I can succeed on my own.

   Practice writing down an important message you'd like to express to someone:

   _____

   _____

   _____

   _____

   _____

   _____

2. **Approach others with a calm, open, and direct manner.** Be ready and willing to engage in a dialogue (that is, a two-way conversation) rather than a monologue (a one-sided conversation).

   Example: "Mom and Dad, can I talk with you about my school assignments? I know it's important for you to be involved, but I feel like I can take on

continued ▶

more responsibility than you're giving me right now. Can we think through this together?"

Practice how you can turn your answer from #1 into a dialogue. What input can you use from the other person's point of view?

_____

_____

_____

_____

_____

_____

3. **Actively listen.** After you've expressed an idea, pay close attention to the other person's response. What message are they trying to express? Clarify either verbally or nonverbally that you understand them.

   Examples: "I get it." "I see what you're saying." "It sounds like you mean . . ." "I hear you."

   Practice some phrases you can use to show the other person you are actively listening:

   _____

   _____

   _____

   _____

   _____

   _____

4. **Use "I" statements.** Focus your statements on your own thoughts, feelings, and experiences, rather than on blaming the other person. You can reframe statements about the other person into an "I" statement, like this:

Examples:

- *You are so unfair. → I think this is unfair.*

- *You are wrong. → I don't agree.*

- *You don't care. → I feel ignored.*

Practice by flipping these sentences to "I" statements:

- *You never listen to me. →* _____

- *You make me so angry. →* _____

- *You're not helping me at all. →* _____

5. **Validate.** Try your best to understand the other person's thoughts, feelings, and experiences. Validation does not mean you have to agree, it simply means that you understand where they are coming from. The more validation you offer to others, the more you will get in return.

Example: "Dad, I understand you want to stay on top of my grades to make sure I succeed. Mom, I get that you give me so many reminders to make sure I don't forget anything. I appreciate that you are both trying to support me."

Practice validation by taking someone else's point of view on a disagreement you've had:

_____

_____

_____

_____

_____

Next, we'll talk about working together to find new solutions to a conflict or problem.

ACTIVITY 21:

Problem-Solving by Working It Out Together

In school, you may have learned a basic problem-solving strategy that includes identifying the problem, brainstorming solutions, choosing one solution to put into action, and then evaluating the outcome.

You already know from part 1 that our brains are solving real-world problems 24/7. Even the simple thought "I'm hungry!" comes with an analysis of ways to solve that problem (looking in the fridge, grabbing an apple, and so on).

Slowing down to be mindful about your problem-solving abilities can help you feel more in control, less stressed, more confident about your chosen solution, and more flexible with trying a different solution, if necessary. Collaborating with others to solve problems can be an even more powerful skill.

Take another look at activity 19: Defining Your Needs (page 58), where you placed a star next to the most important need you'd like to assert right now. Think through how you might brainstorm solutions. Use the following prompts to organize your thoughts:

1. What is the problem?

    Example: I feel responsible enough to get good grades with less of my parents' involvement. My mom and dad are concerned that if they step back, my grades might slip.

    _____

    _____

    _____

2. Brainstorm every possible solution and jot everything down without judgment.

    Example: We could keep things as they are; my parents could totally leave it to me; my dad can check the parent portal less often; my mom could give me fewer reminders about assignments that are due.

    _____

    _____

    _____

3. Choose one solution to try out.

Example: My parents reduce their involvement over the next two weeks as a "trial period."

_____

_____

_____

4. Devise a plan to take action.

Example: My dad will check the parent portal only once per week; my mom will give me only one reminder about assignments that are due the following day. If my grades stay the same over the next two weeks, they will reduce their involvement a bit more.

_____

_____

_____

5. Evaluate the solution and revise if necessary.

Example: My grades stayed the same in all classes, and even got better in one class. So, my parents have agreed to give me more autonomy with my school-work for the rest of this grading period.

_____

_____

_____

ACTIVITY 22: Focusing on Others

Another technique to reduce stress is to shine the spotlight on others' needs. Noticing other people's challenges and helping other people, even in small ways, can make a big difference in your own perspective.

Research has shown that contributing to other people, to your community, or to the world has many benefits, like feeling a greater sense of purpose, gaining a broader perspective, and raising your self-esteem and confidence. When we become overwhelmed with stress, we can start to feel like we've lost our direction. Focusing on helping others rewards us with a sense of pride, purpose, and potential.

Your problems might seem smaller when compared to other people's. Or you might learn a new way of handling a problem that you hadn't thought of before. Learning new skills and using those skills to serve others in need is a surefire way to feel good about yourself and take a break from your own stress and worries.

Your contributions don't need to be huge to be meaningful. Look through this list and check off some things you can try over the next few days to help another person. Feel free to add your own original ideas using the blank write-in lines, too:

☐ Help your family: Pitch in with chores like cooking, cleaning, or taking care of siblings—take on more responsibility to take it off someone else's plate.

☐ Help your peers: Give more compliments, motivate others to succeed in their own pursuits, or recognize when a classmate needs a helping hand.

☐ Help out in your local community: Take the lead in a school club, sport, or activity, help organize fundraisers, or offer your help to teachers and coaches.

☐ Help out in your larger community: Look into volunteer organizations like the YMCA, Boys and Girls Club, or other national organizations to find opportunities to help your community.

☐ _____

☐ _____

☐ _____

ACTIVITY 23: Embracing Gratitude

Taking time to practice gratitude or appreciation for what you have in your life right now can immediately shift you out of a stressed state. Some things to practice gratitude toward might be: you and your loved ones' health; relationships you cherish; having basic necessities like food, shelter, and clothing; and the successes you've enjoyed so far in your life.

The following ideas can remind you to practice gratitude more often, at least once every day. Place a checkmark next to ideas that you are interested in trying. Feel free to add your own original ideas using the blank write-in lines, too:

☐ Journal. Write or draw three things you are grateful for today. Try to add new things each day.

☐ Create a gratitude jar or box. Jot down words of gratitude on small slips of paper that you add to your jar/box, and watch it fill up over time.

☐ Take time to experience and appreciate the things you're grateful for. For example, if you're grateful for access to nature, take time for a walk, spend time gardening, or simply sit outside.

☐ Compose a letter. Write a letter or email to someone—a family member, friend, romantic partner, teacher, coach, or other person—describing what you appreciate about your relationship with them. You can choose to send it or simply save it for yourself.

☐ Create a collage. Collect pictures, words, and mementos to create a visual representation of the people and things in your life for which you are grateful. Hang it somewhere you will see it every day.

☐ Meditate. During a meditation exercise, try focusing on one or two people or things for which you are grateful. Concentrate on an image that helps you feel content, calm, and peaceful.

☐ _____

☐ _____

☐ _____

ACTIVITY 24: Tuning In to Your Thoughts

Shifting your perspective from stress to gratitude or to helping others is an example of "reframing." This is a technique used in cognitive behavioral therapy (CBT), a helpful form of therapy that helps us realize that our thoughts, emotions, and behaviors are all interconnected.

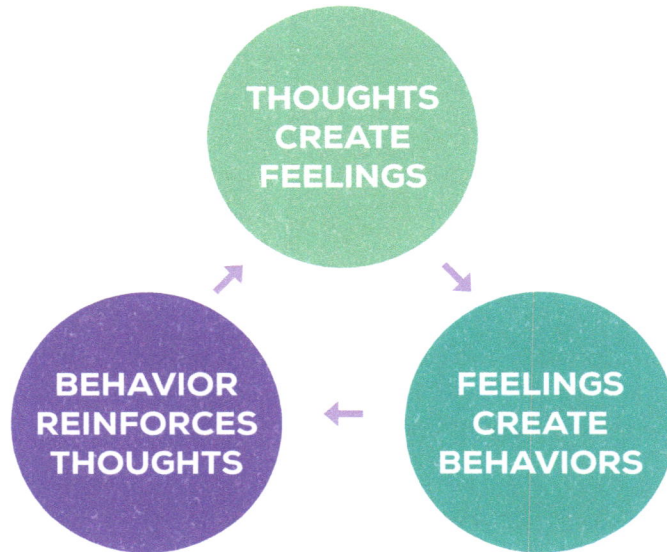

Let's say you often feel nervous about raising your hand in class. Your automatic thought might be, "I think I know the answer, but I'm not 100 percent sure. If I mess it up, my teacher will think I'm dumb and my classmates will probably make fun of me." Naturally, this makes you feel anxious (9 out of 10), so you decide not to raise your hand.

Now, imagine the same scenario, but with a different thought that makes you feel less anxious and more confident about raising your hand. What might a more helpful thought be?

_____

_____

HINT: *One possibility is "I think I know the answer, but I'm not 100 percent sure. I might mess it up. But this teacher knows I'm a good student. And even if my classmates laugh for a minute, they'll forget about it by the end of class." This thought could cause your anxiety to drop to 5 out of 10, giving you just enough confidence to raise your hand.*

Let's take a closer look at how CBT can help reduce stress.

ACTIVITY 25: Noticing My Common Thinking Mistakes

While people often notice an emotion first, such as a rush of anger, CBT asserts that a thought already has passed through your mind, *causing* that emotion. If you've ever felt instantly nervous or jittery just at the sight of your crush, it's likely that your mind was already thinking, "This person is special to me, and I care about what they think of me."

Like with ACT, a main concept in CBT is that *thoughts are just thoughts, not facts*. Learning to slow down, check our thoughts, and challenge the thinking mistakes that pop up can keep us in control of how we feel and act.

Here are some common thinking mistakes. Check off ones that you've noticed yourself thinking before, then try to catch yourself when these unhelpful thoughts pop up during times of stress:

☐ **All-or-nothing thinking:** thinking in extremes and missing or discounting the gray area in between.

Example: Either I get an A in this class, or I've totally failed.

☐ **Mind reading:** assuming you know what people are thinking, without real evidence.

Example: She hasn't said anything, but I'm sure my coach thinks I'm the worst player on the team.

☐ **Fortune-telling:** predicting the future, as if it is certain.

Example: My mom will say no when I ask her if I can go to this party, so why bother asking?

☐ **Catastrophizing:** believing that your worst-case scenario will happen, and you won't be able to tolerate it.

Example: If I bring this up with my partner, what if it starts an argument? What if they get mad at me? What if we can't resolve the fight? What if we break up?

☐ **Negative filter/discounting the positives:** focusing only on the negatives of a situation and not paying attention to the positives.

Example: We were having a really good time on this date, until I said something so stupid at the end. Now they think I'm a loser.

☐ **Should-ing:** judging and guilting yourself (or others) according to rigid rules about how things "should" be.

Examples: I shouldn't have made so many mistakes while practicing my instrument.

ACTIVITY 26: Catch It, Check It, Correct It

CBT exercises often include a thought record that helps slow down our thinking so we can catch our automatic thoughts, check for any thinking mistakes, and correct our thoughts to more helpful, accurate ones.

Read the example thought record first. Then think of your own example of a recent stressful situation. Fill out a row of the thought record based on your own experience using your new skills to Catch It, Check It, and Correct It.

SITUATION What is happening?	EMOTIONS What are you feeling? How strongly, from 0 to 10?	THOUGHTS What are you thinking?			EMOTIONS Re-rate your emotions now.
		CATCH IT What thought is going through your mind?	**CHECK IT** Is this thought true? Are there any thinking mistakes?	**CORRECT IT** What's a more accurate, helpful thought?	
I'm home alone on a Saturday, bored, scrolling social media	Lonely 10 Sad 8 Jealous 8	It seems like everyone else has more fun, more friends, and no stress.	No. I'm using a negative filter and telling myself I "should" be out on a Saturday.	I have two good friends, and we just went out last week and had a great time. Plus, I know other people have stress, too.	Lonely 5 Sad 4 Jealous 4

ACTIVITY 27: Challenging My "Worst-Case Worry"

Another CBT technique is to take on catastrophizing thoughts head-on. Instead of letting yourself spiral into "what if?" territory, this technique can root you back into actually realizing what your "worst case" worry represents and just how likely it is to actually come true. To begin, ask yourself these three questions:

1. What is the worst-case scenario that I fear?

2. How likely is the worst-case scenario to happen?

3. If it does happen, will I be able to survive it?

Read the example first. Then think of your own example of a recent stressful situation. Fill out answers to each of the three questions. Chances are that you'll realize your situation, and your "worst-case worry," isn't nearly as life-or-death as it might seem at first.

Stressful situation	What is the worst-case scenario that I fear?	How likely will the worst-case scenario happen?	Even if it does happen, will I be able to survive it?
My partner and I are arguing a lot lately, more than ever before.	What if they decide to break up with me? They might leave me and start dating someone else. I'll never have another relationship like this.	Feels like 50 percent. We've had times like this in the past when we argued a lot and we've never broken up. So, maybe more like a 25 percent chance.	I would be heartbroken. I'd feel devastated. It would be really hard to show up to school or hang out without them. I'd cry for weeks! But yes, I would survive. I've been through a breakup before, and I know it gets better with time.

ACTIVITY 28: Facing My Fears

One last way that CBT can help reduce anxiety and stress focuses on changing your behaviors. It's a fairly simple shift that can then create healthier thoughts and more positive feelings.

"Exposure" is the CBT term we use for pushing yourself outside your comfort zone to face a stressful situation. The more often you engage in exposure (instead of avoidance), the more confidence you will build and the less stress or anxiety you will feel. A "fear hierarchy" or "fear ladder" helps you think through small steps you can take to reach your goal of conquering a fear or stressor.

Read the example first. Then, think of your own example of a fearful situation that you've avoided in the past. Fill out your own small steps toward reaching your greater goal. Start with the "least scary" steps at the bottom, working your way up to the bigger steps at the top.

Go to a bigger party for an hour with friends.

The fear I am facing is:

showing up to a party and making small talk with people.

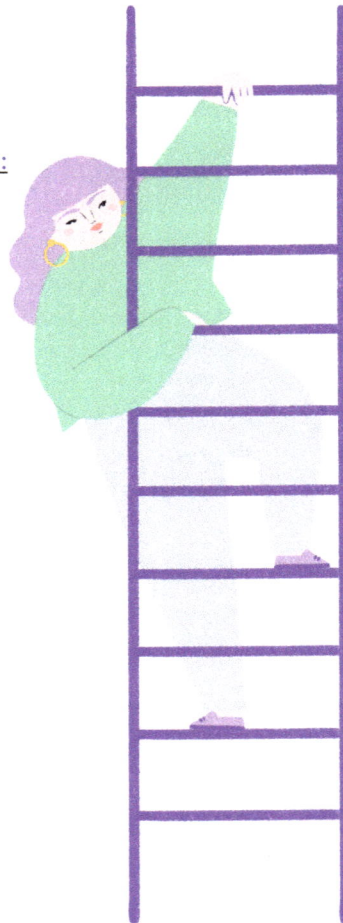

Go to a small gathering for 30 minutes.

Practice holding longer conversations with my friends.

Ask an acquaintance a broad question, like "How was your weekend?"

Practice smiling or giving an "up nod" to my classmates.

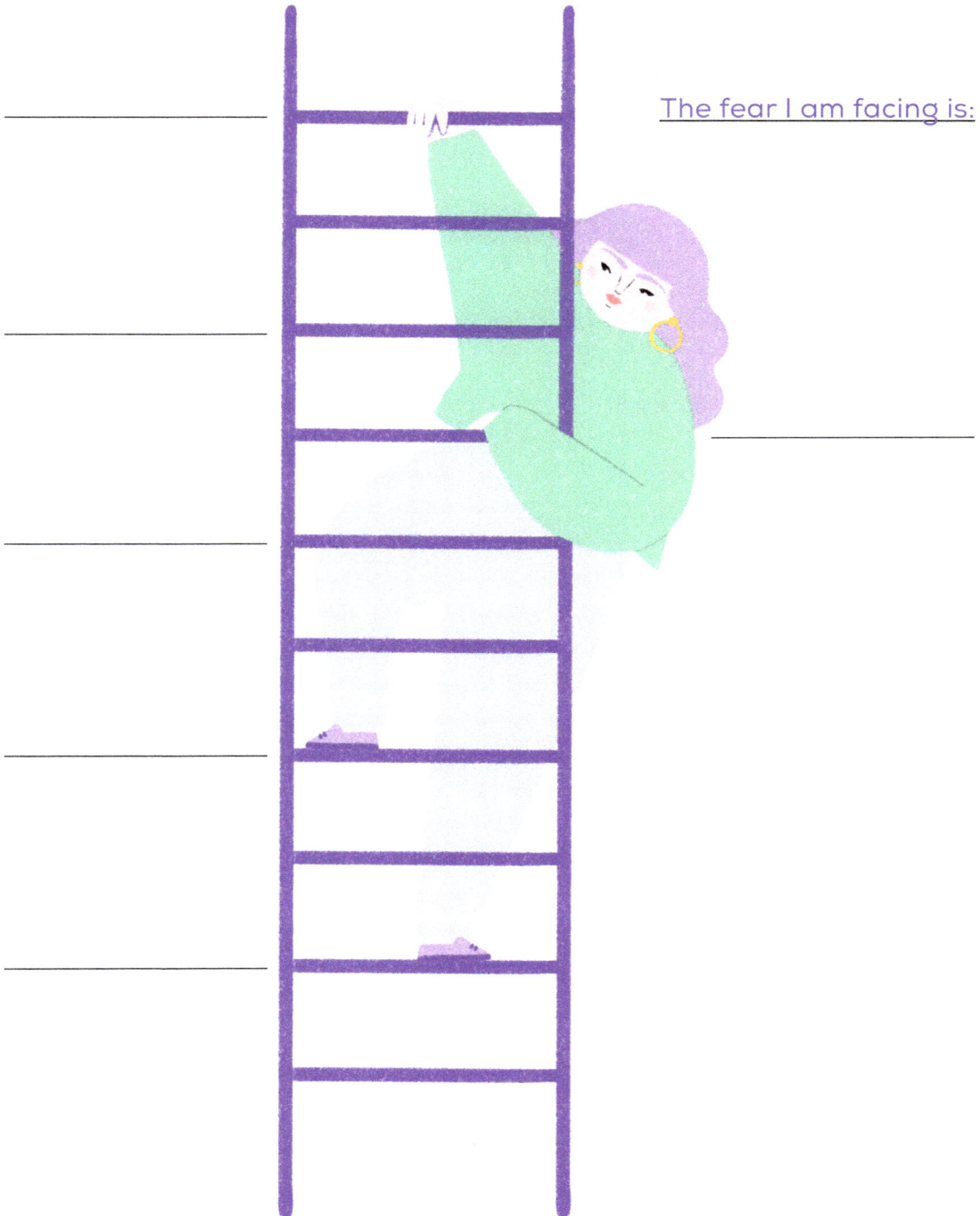

The fear I am facing is:

ACTIVITY 29: Live It to Learn It

Exposure exercises are especially helpful in building *resilience*, the ability to recover from difficult things. Resilience is not something you're born with; it's something you learn.

The following chart lists 10 characteristics or resources that make people resilient. Read each trait and decide if it's true about you or not. Place a checkmark in the correct column. Then, write down a time when you drew on that resource.

Resilient Trait	Yes, this is true about me	No, I need to improve on this	Write about a time you used this trait
Sample trait: Resourcefulness	✓		Last week's group project was pretty disorganized. After our first planning session, I created a group calendar to share with each person's tasks and deadlines. Everything got done a day early!
1. **Curiosity and enthusiasm for learning:** I like to learn and master new skills.			
2. **Perseverance:** I can commit to personal goals I set for myself.			
3. **Action-oriented:** My sense of control helps me take positive action steps toward my goals.			
4. **Realistic thinking:** I know the limits to my control, and I can let go of things that are out of my control.			

Resilient Trait	Yes, this is true about me	No, I need to improve on this	Write about a time you used this trait
5. **Pride:** I celebrate my successes and try not to dwell on mistakes.			
6. **Patience:** I can tolerate the uncomfortable feeling of waiting for a difficult situation to pass with time.			
7. **Sense of humor:** I always try to find something to laugh about, even in the worst of times.			
8. **Flexibility:** I'm confident I can adapt to changes in my life, even if it's not easy.			
9. **Optimism:** I try to keep a positive attitude, even when things are hard.			
10. **Social support:** I have close attachments to family, friends, and others that I can depend on.			

ACTIVITY 30: Revisiting Mindfulness

One final form of therapy that is very helpful in stress reduction is dialectical behavior therapy (DBT). In a way, DBT combines ACT and CBT theories to teach the skills needed to build what DBT's creator calls a "life worth living." "Dialectic" refers to two opposites that can coexist at the same time, for example, believing "I am proud of myself *and* there are some things I am working to improve." We'll discuss five parts of DBT that are especially helpful for teens managing stress. The first is mindfulness.

Although we've discussed aspects of mindfulness, DBT adds an important element to it. Beyond bringing awareness to your present moment, DBT mindfulness exercises encourage you to notice your thoughts, feelings, and physical sensations, all *without judgment*. Thus, the goal is not to clear your mind, but just to tune in to it. Let observations come, acknowledge them, and release them. There's no need to judge a feeling, try to change it, or try to solve a problem. Simply notice the thought float by as if it were on a cloud and stay tuned to the next thought that approaches.

Take a minute now to tune in to your thoughts. Jot them down as you simply observe your train of thought.

_____

_____

_____

_____

_____

_____

ACTIVITY 31: My Stress Journal

Ready for a bit of a break between all of your stress-busting work? Journaling can help clear your mind, release emotions that build up over time, clarify how to solve a problem, and increase your self-awareness.

You might find the idea of starting your journal scary or just too much, but here's the truth: there are tons of unique ways to journal—you don't even have to use words. There are no rules for expressing yourself in a safe, private space. Circle some ways you might use the pages of your journal:

- Write
- Jot down words or phrases
- Make bulleted lists
- Draw
- Doodle
- Try writing different personal mantras
- Write a poem

- Write out song lyrics
- Write letters to people (no need to share)
- Write a pro and con list
- Write a to-do list
- Make a bucket list for the month, season, or year
- Write out a prayer

If blank pages feel too hard to start with, you can also research journaling prompts online, which offer ideas such as:

- Write about what you did today. Include the best parts and the most challenging parts of your day.

- Describe or draw a calm, peaceful scene that helps you relax when you imagine it. Include details about what you see, hear, smell, feel, and taste within this scene.

- List three people you feel grateful to have in your life. Explain why.

- Write about what scares you. Have your fears changed over time?

Keep your stress journal handy for any moment when your stress starts to get the better of you. Now, let's explore more about DBT together.

ACTIVITY 32: Walking the Middle Path with Wise Mind

Creating balance is a central idea in DBT. Much like correcting "all-or-nothing" thinking, walking the middle path encourages you to consider a different perspective. As discussed earlier, "dialectics" refers to two things that seem like opposites but can both be true. Think about the importance of balancing hard work *and* rest, independence *and* social support, or your own sense of self-acceptance *and* self-improvement.

Especially in stressful times when emotions are intense, it can be difficult to choose our actions thoughtfully and carefully. Sometimes, we react quickly and instinctively based on our feelings, without thinking through the consequences. Other times, we might focus solely on "the facts" and not consider the emotional aspects.

Responding to stress requires a balance between considering the facts and also tuning in to your feelings. We call that state of balance your "wise mind." Using your wise mind to solve problems and make decisions means you are considering logic *and* emotion in order to make the most balanced choice possible. Here's an example of making a wise mind decision about attending college:

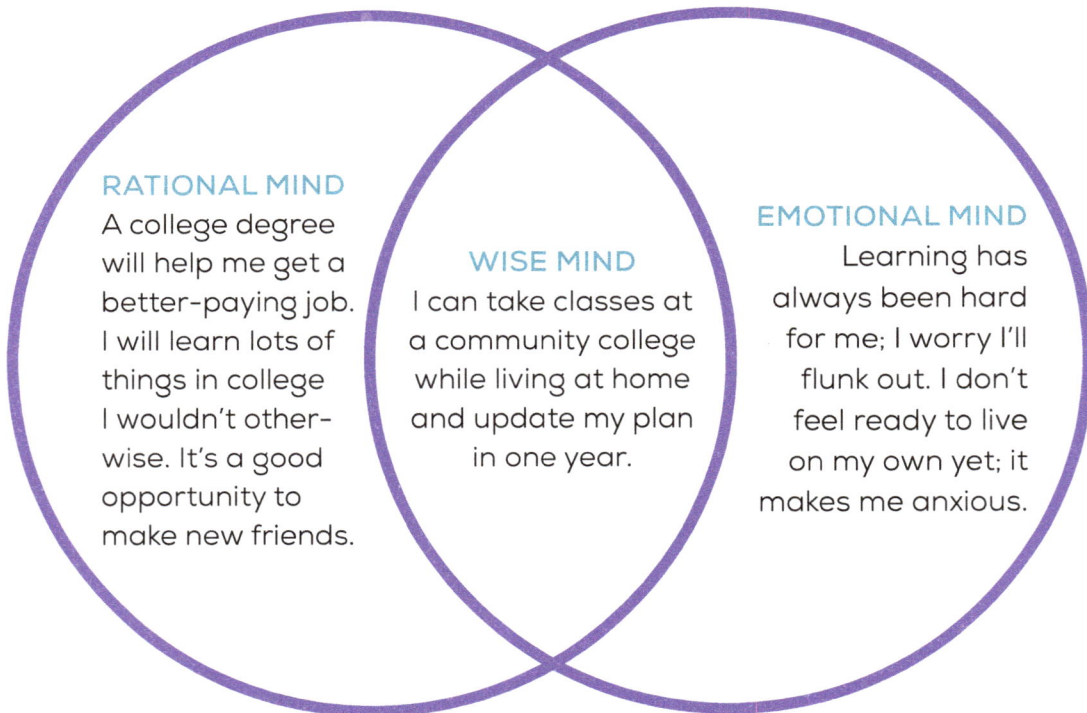

RATIONAL MIND
A college degree will help me get a better-paying job. I will learn lots of things in college I wouldn't otherwise. It's a good opportunity to make new friends.

WISE MIND
I can take classes at a community college while living at home and update my plan in one year.

EMOTIONAL MIND
Learning has always been hard for me; I worry I'll flunk out. I don't feel ready to live on my own yet; it makes me anxious.

Think of a difficult decision you are trying to make in your life right now and fill out the diagram. Under Rational Mind, write the facts about the situation. Under Emotional Mind, write what feelings it brings up for you. In Wise Mind, try to find a balanced resolution.

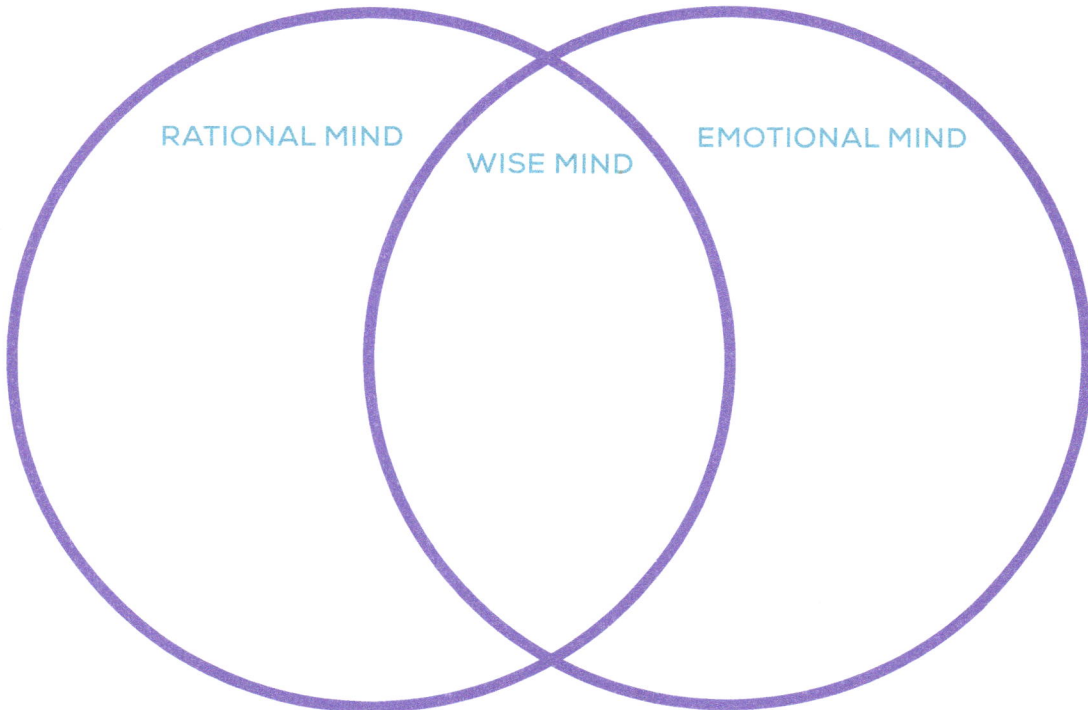

RATIONAL MIND   WISE MIND   EMOTIONAL MIND

ACTIVITY 33: Dealing with Difficult Emotions, DBT Style

DBT teaches different strategies for managing two distinct emotional experiences. Distress tolerance strategies are like survival skills for emotional crisis moments. They're very useful for taking care of yourself when you've reached your emotional breaking point. These are immediate, short-term techniques meant to ground you in the present moment and to temporarily distract you from your overwhelming emotions. Some examples include:

- **Focus on sensations.** Use your five senses to create a safe physical sensation that distracts your mind from overwhelming thoughts and feelings. For example, hold an ice cube in your hand, eat something sour, or draw gently on your forearm with a pen.

- **Push away the stress.** Temporarily stop thinking about the problem by mentally swiping the thoughts away every time they pop up.

- **Engage in an activity.** Shift your focus away from your thoughts and feelings by concentrating on an activity like a hobby, project, or schoolwork.

- **Exercise.** Engage in intense, strenuous exercise like a long run or jumping jacks to get your heart rate up and your oxygen flowing. Push as hard as you can until you're physically exhausted.

Emotional regulation techniques are longer-term strategies for managing the daily emotional ups and downs that come with life so that you can feel more balanced and in control. Some examples include:

- **Accumulate positive experiences.** Build "a life worth living" by increasing positive experiences and pleasant activities in your life. Be sure to include things that give you a sense of accomplishment.

- **Ride the wave.** Look at your feelings like a wave washing over you. You can't stop it or control it. So, instead of trying to push the feeling away or trying to hold on to it, simply ride the wave until it passes.

- **Create the opposite emotion.** If you're feeling sad, watch a movie that makes you laugh. If you're feeling nervous, listen to soothing music that relaxes you.

Look through this list of ideas and check off ones that would be helpful for you with each emotional experience:

Idea	This could help temporarily distract me from an emotional crisis.	This could help me manage my emotions on a day-to-day basis.
Watch my favorite movie		
Go for a walk		
Take a shower or bath		
Listen to music		
Cook and/or enjoy my favorite meal		
Engage in/learn a new hobby		
Spend time with a family member		
Call, text, or video chat a friend		
Journal/write		
Pray or meditate		
Draw or doodle		
Drink some water		
Splash cold water on my face		
Count to 10		
Use a fidget spinner		
Focus on deep breathing		
Practice a mindfulness exercise		
Visualize a calm, peaceful scene		
Use progressive muscle relaxation		
Stretch		
Exercise		

ACTIVITY 34: Dealing with Stressful Situations, DBT Style

DBT teaches us skills to help improve our ability to interact with other people. This can reduce a lot of stress that comes from conflicts, arguments, and disagreements with others.

We've already discussed some techniques for asserting your needs, communicating effectively, and problem-solving with others. One more skill that's very important to know is how to handle conflicts with others, like when you have an argument with a parent or friend.

Take a moment to remember a recent argument, disagreement, or conflict you've had with someone, when you noticed your emotional thermometer (page 42) rising with anger, frustration, or indignation. Once you've got that firmly in your mind, try practicing the THINK technique:

Think about the situation from the other person's perspective. Put yourself in the other person's shoes and try to figure out how they see the situation.

_____

_____

_____

Have empathy. Imagine the other person's feelings. Are they also angry? Frustrated? Feeling disrespected? Hurt? Sad?

_____

_____

_____

Interpretations. Brainstorm other interpretations or explanations for the person's behavior. You probably have already made an assumption about why they acted a certain way. Now, try to think of other possible reasons.

_____

_____

_____

Notice the other person. Stop for a moment and pay attention to their actions now. Are they making an effort to improve the situation? Are they showing that they care? Are they struggling with their own stressful feelings?

_____

_____

_____

Kindness. Move forward with a kind approach. This doesn't necessarily mean forgive and forget, or to give up in a passive way. This simply means treat the other person in a respectful way or the same way you wish to be treated. You might say something like, "I'm feeling too upset right now to fix this problem. Right now, I need space, and we can figure this out together later on."

_____

_____

_____

ACTIVITY 35: My Self-Care Plan

At the beginning of part 2, we looked at the self-care wheel (page 27) as a way to think about taking care of yourself in different ways. And whether you realized it or not, all of the activities presented in part 2 fit into one of the six categories that make up the self-care wheel: mental health, physical health, creativity/spirituality, relationships, environment, and personal growth.

Now that you've learned new techniques, let's take some time to add more details into your self-care wheel. In each piece of the wheel, add three new ideas, strategies, or skills you will start working on to reduce stress.

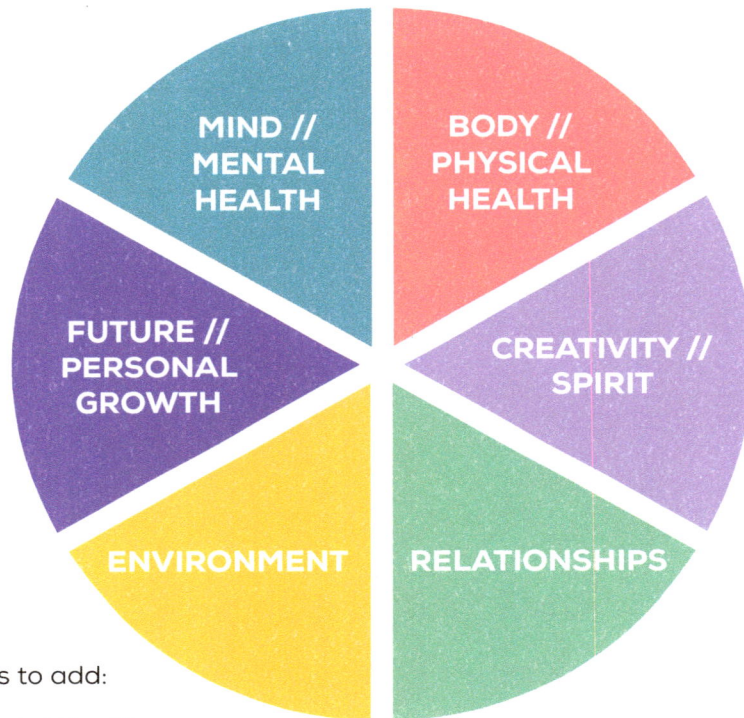

Examples to add:

1. Mind/Mental Health

   - I will start practicing visualization at bedtime every night.

   - I will try to catch my negative "thinking mistakes" and correct them.

   - I will start trying to make decisions using my "wise mind."

   _____

   _____

   _____

2. Body/Physical Health

- I will practice deep breathing, especially when I notice my stress ther-mometer is getting up to a 5.

- I will start going to bed 30 minutes earlier each night.

- I will make time to skateboard three times a week.

_____

_____

_____

3. Creativity/Spirituality

- I will start practicing mindfulness when I feel stressed by soothing my five senses.

- To help me relax, I'll learn to play a song on the ukulele.

- I will examine what other feelings are beneath the surface whenever I notice my anger thermometer rising.

_____

_____

_____

4. Relationships

- I will make an effort to be less passive and more assertive about my needs.

- I will remember to use the THINK method when I need to resolve a conflict with someone.

- I will face my fears and attend the next party I'm invited to.

_____

_____

_____

continued ▶

5. Environment

- I will add three things I'm grateful for to my journal each week.

- I'll wash the dinner dishes three nights a week to take pressure off my family members.

- I will ask my family to sign up for a volunteer activity with me to help our community.

_____

_____

_____

6. Future/Personal Growth

- I will use my journal to brainstorm action steps to help me live according to my top three values.

- I will ask for help from my big sister/guidance counselor with my college applications, so I don't feel so overwhelmed.

- I will keep working on building resilient traits (like taking pride in my successes and being flexible).

_____

_____

_____

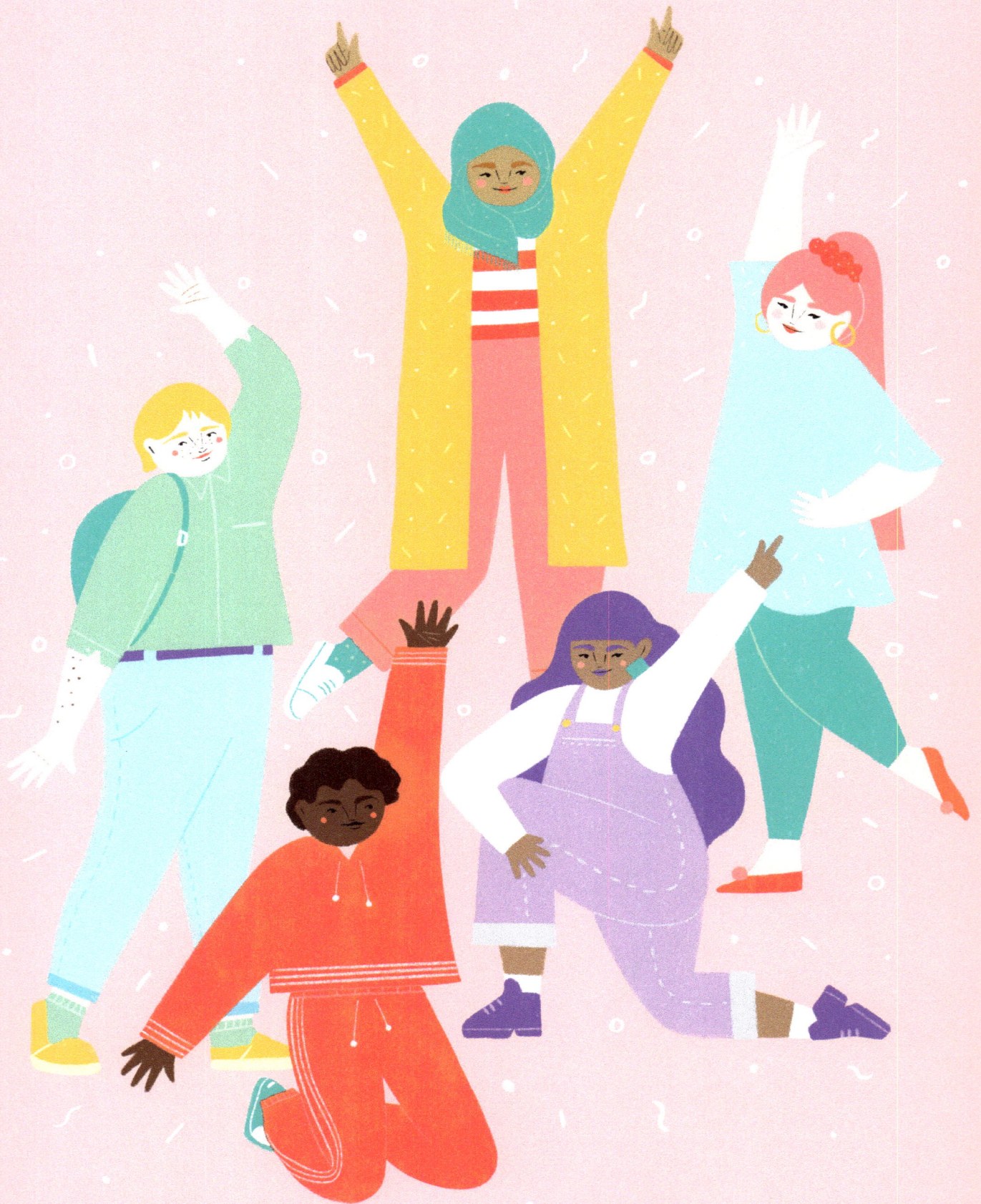

PART 3

Teen Talk: Your Real Questions Answered

Part 1 of this workbook provided you with a solid under-standing of stress and how it affects both your mind and body, as well as an introduction to a variety of stress-reducing techniques. Part 2 helped you practice specific stress-reducing skills to find those that work for you. In part 3, we'll explore together how to apply these new techniques to real-life situations that commonly cause stress, thus becoming less stressed in these moments and the calmest we can be.

I Have a Question About Stress and . . .

continued ▸

I HAVE A QUESTION ABOUT STRESS AND . . .

Self-Care When I'm Overwhelmed

Q: My life gets so busy sometimes that I feel like I have no downtime when I can just talk to my friends or chill out on my own. This happens every fall—keeping up with school, playing sports, and getting involved in after-school activities just feels like too much to handle. How can I even fit in self-care when I'm so exhausted?

A: I hear you! So many teens feel overscheduled and exhausted these days. It seems like you're tuned in to your body and mind, so that you're aware of when your stress thermometer is starting to rise.

Let's take an acceptance and commitment therapy (ACT) approach to this question. Ask yourself:

What is in my control right now?

_____

_____

_____

Which activities are the most meaningful to me that I want to focus my energy on?

_____

_____

_____

With that in mind, review your fall schedule. Is every activity necessary? Is there something you can cut or postpone?

_____

_____

_____

If you can cut back, great! Use that time you've just added back into your schedule for relaxing and pleasurable activities (like doing absolutely nothing!). If not, then your focus might be on building up resiliency that will carry you through another fall season. What do you need to be able to sustain the amount of energy and focus required of you for those couple of months?

Also, try to shift your thinking from "self-care is an extra activity to squeeze in" to "self-care helps me perform at my best, both mentally and physically." These busy times are exactly when self-care strategies are most important. Getting enough sleep and eating healthy meals will supply you with the stamina you need for a long day. Closing your eyes and focusing on deep breathing for five minutes between activities can clear your mind and shift your focus. Listening to a guided meditation podcast before bed can help create a restful, relaxed state of mind that helps you drift off to sleep.

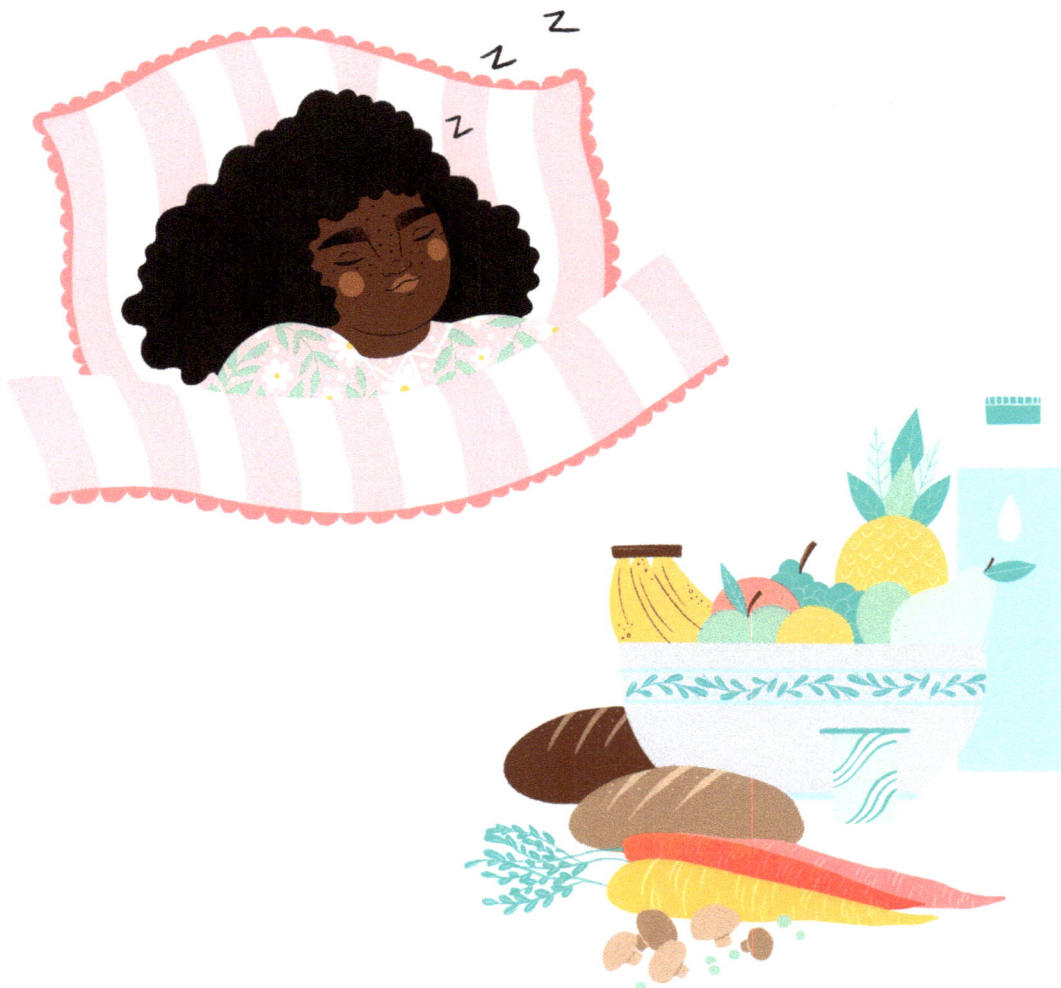

I HAVE A QUESTION ABOUT STRESS AND . . .

Handling Tests and Exams

Q: I'm a pretty good student, but I've always had a hard time taking tests. I get so nervous and freaked out about failing that my mind goes blank, and I struggle to show the knowledge that I really have. It's always been frustrating, but now I'm preparing to take standardized tests. I'm really worried that I'm going to fail miserably and mess up my chances for college. How can I stop stressing so much about tests?

A: Feeling anxious about tests is a really common experience for teens, mostly because there's a lot of pressure to succeed on every assignment, every exam, and every report card. If this happens on all your tests over a long period of time, and it's so severe that it negatively affects your performance, it might be a case of test-taking anxiety. Here are three strategies to try:

- Take care of yourself before the test. Make sure you get a good night's sleep, eat a healthy breakfast, and use some self-soothing strategies as the test approaches (listen to your favorite music, talk with a friend to distract you, write in your journal about how you're feeling).

- Use the cognitive behavioral therapy (CBT) strategy of "catch, check, and correct," which we discussed in activity 26 (page 68). Catch the negative thoughts that are running through your mind, like "I'm going to fail miserably and mess up my chances for college." That's an example of a thinking mistake (catastrophizing) that is working against you. Instead, try to shift your thoughts to a confidence-boosting mantra, such as "I'm smart. I'm a good student. I studied hard. I know everything I need to know to pass this test."

- Practice your "crisis skills" ahead of time, like what we learned in activity 33 (page 78), so they are ready when you need them. Practice deep breathing, focus on your five senses, and visualize a successful test-taking experience following a script like this one:

I envision entering the testing room with confidence, taking a comfortable seat, and receiving the test. My nerves make me feel a bit excited, but I steady my breathing. I see myself reading the first question and feeling confident that I am prepared to succeed. I imagine myself selecting the correct answers, at a pace that feels right to me. I see myself finishing the test on time, feeling satisfied and content with my performance.

Try writing your own visualization script:

_____

_____

_____

_____

_____

_____

_____

_____

_____

_____

_____

I HAVE A QUESTION ABOUT STRESS AND . . .

Trying to Be Perfect

Q: As I get older, it feels like there's more and more pressure to be perfect. I have to get good grades, be involved in clubs, play an instrument, volunteer—all the things that will look good on a college application. My parents expect me to be on the honor roll, and my teachers say I have "so much potential." I've noticed I even put pressure on myself. How do I stop wanting to be perfect?

A: I'm really impressed that you've noticed the stress you are feeling and started to figure out where it's coming from. Expectations are really high and come from every direction. Of course, parents and teachers hope for the best for you—a good education, a great future job, and happiness! But that can feel like pressure to get everything right all day, every day, as if being perfect is the only way to achieve these dreams. And let's be honest: nobody is perfect. Take a moment to confront the fear of *not* being perfect.

Try the three-question exercise from activity 27 that helps you challenge your "worst-case worry" (page 69):

Stressful situation	What is the worst-case scenario that I fear?	How likely is it that the worst-case scenario will happen?	Even if it does happen, will I be able to survive it?

The truth is probably that your worst-case scenario is unlikely. This kind of thinking can help you adjust your outlook so that instead of fretting about being perfect—which no one can achieve—you're shooting for "my best" with the knowledge that you'll be able to handle multiple outcomes. Talk to your parents and teachers; I'm sure they can agree that what's most important is that you are putting forth your best effort.

Bonus: it's much easier to feel good about yourself if that's how you are measuring your success.

I HAVE A QUESTION ABOUT STRESS AND . . .

Feeling Lonely

Q: I've been feeling lonely because I don't have any real, close friends. I talk to a couple of kids at school, and I have a bunch of online friends that I game with, but it's really hard for me to talk to people face-to-face. I guess I'm shy, but I worry so much about other people liking me that I get too nervous to just have a normal conversation. It seems like everyone else has tons of friends, and I feel really bad about myself when I see social media posts of other kids hanging out together. How do I get over this shyness and insecurity?

A: I'm sorry to hear you've been feeling lonely. A lot of teens feel the same way, even those posting pictures with big smiles on social media who seem like they have thousands of friends! I would suggest you try to focus less on those posts and more on the goals you have set for yourself: having easier face-to-face conversations, making more friends, and enjoying a social life of your own.

The quickest way to get started is to make a fear ladder (introduced in activity 28 on page 70), detailing a hierarchy of your fears:

"really hard" = ask a friend to hang out after school
"medium" = sit next to a friendly classmate in class
"easy" = having conversations online

Fill in the steps in between these levels of difficulty and challenge yourself every day to go outside your comfort zone by moving up one small step. I bet you'll start to see a positive change in how others respond to you, which can help you feel more confident to move up to the next step.

Ask a friend to hang
out after school.

_____

_____

_____

Sit next to a friendly
classmate in class.

_____

_____

_____

Having
conversations online.

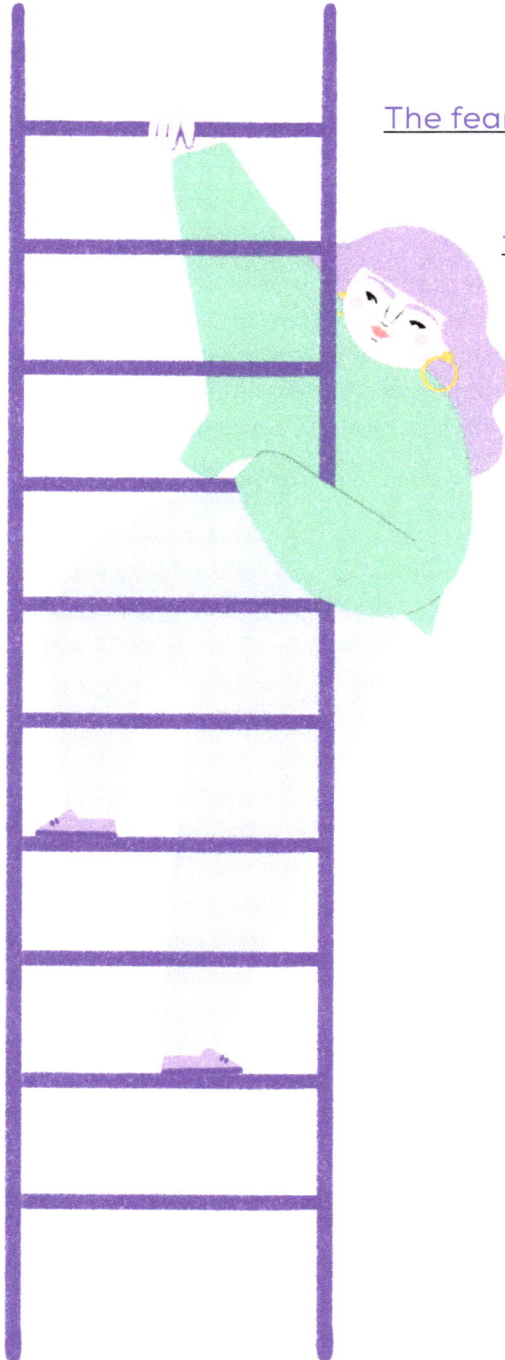

_____

The fear I am facing is:

feeling lonely.

I HAVE A QUESTION ABOUT STRESS AND . . .

Feeling Left Out

Q: Over this past summer, my best friend and I didn't get to spend much time together because we were both busy with camp, sports, and other things. Now that school has started, he's still acting distant. We don't have any classes together, and I see him spending a lot of time with other friends. They're gaming together and posting social media photos of hangouts that I'm not invited to. I'm really hurt and sad, because it seems like he's outgrown our friendship. What should I do?

A: It's true that friendships change over time, especially from one school year to the next, and this can be very stressful. It's important to try your best to communicate with your friend and make sure you have all the facts. Believing he doesn't want to be friends with you anymore is an assumption—it might be true, but it just as easily might be a misinterpretation.

Use these communication strategies (introduced in activity 20 on page 59) to start an honest conversation:

a. Collect your thoughts. What message are you trying to send? What is important for your friend to know? It may help to write this in a journal, or even compose a letter to him to help you organize your thoughts.

_____

_____

_____

_____

_____

_____

b. Approach your friend in a calm, open, and direct manner. Be ready and willing to engage in a dialogue (a two-way conversation) rather than a monologue (a one-sided conversation). You might start with "I wanted to talk with you about something. It feels like we're not as close as we used to be, and I miss hanging out with you. Have you noticed?" Try to come up with a conversation opener here:

_____

_____

_____

_____

c. Actively listen. After you've expressed your thoughts and feelings, pay close attention to your friend's response. Pay attention to the message he is trying to express and clarify that you understand him. Use verbal and/or nonverbal cues to show you are listening.

d. Use "I" statements. Focus your statements on your own thoughts, feelings, and experiences, without blaming your friend. For example:

- Instead of "You've been ignoring me," you can say, "I've been feeling left out."

- Instead of "You're acting cold," you can say, "I'm sad that we're not as close as we used to be."

- Instead of "It's obvious you don't want to be friends anymore," you can say, "I wonder if our friendship is still important to you."

e. Validate. Try your best to understand your friend's thoughts, feelings, and experience. Validation does not mean you have to agree; it simply means that you understand where he is coming from. For example, he may want to expand his friendship circle right now, and so he's spending time with new friends. While it may be hurtful, can you understand his point of view?

Once you've talked with your friend and have more accurate information, then you can make a "wise mind" decision with less emotional stress and more self-assuredness. Your next steps might be choosing to work on strengthening your friendship and/or exploring new friendships of your own.

I HAVE A QUESTION ABOUT STRESS AND . . .

A Friendship

Q: I have a friend who I've known since we were little kids. The problem is, they always seem to have some kind of crisis going on. When we were younger, I was happy to listen, but I'm getting tired of the one-sided friendship. They never ask how I'm doing, and they make everything about them. I do worry that they need help, but I can't always handle the added stress. What should I do?

A: It's clear that you are a compassionate person who cares about helping others. As you get older, it starts to become clearer that your own needs are important, too! Any relationship, including friendships, require a healthy balance of give-and-take. You need to lean on them sometimes, too.

First, you should know that it's not your responsibility to take care of them the same way a parent or a therapist would. I would encourage you to talk to a trusted adult (like your own parent, a teacher, a coach, a religious leader) who can get them the support they need.

Then, try talking to them about your feelings. Try out the easy-to-remember THINK acronym from activity 34 (page 80) to try and resolve this conflict:

- **T**hink about the situation from their perspective. Put yourself in their shoes and try to figure out how they see the situation. (Do they even realize you have these feelings?)

- **H**ave empathy. Imagine their feelings. (Are they going through a difficult time right now?)

- **I**nterpretations. Brainstorm other interpretations, or explanations, for their behavior. (Do they notice that they monopolize every conversation?)

- **N**otice the other person. Stop for a moment and pay attention to their actions now. Are they making an effort to improve the situation? Are they showing that they care?

- **K**indness. Move forward with a kind approach. This doesn't necessarily mean forgive and forget, or to give up in a passive way. This simply means treat the other person in a respectful way (the same way you wish to be treated). You might say something like, "I try really hard to be a good friend to you, and I really wish you could offer me some support, too."

Then, based on how they respond to you asserting your own needs, you can make an informed decision to work on building a more balanced friendship or to refocus your efforts on healthier friendships that meet your needs.

I HAVE A QUESTION ABOUT STRESS AND . . .
Dating

Q: I feel sort of stuck when it comes to dating. On one hand, I really want to start dating and maybe even be in a relationship. On the other hand, I feel super nervous about it, and I can't even bring myself to flirt with my crush because it's so embarrassing. I think I'm also nervous about the idea of getting physical. Is it normal to feel confused about this?

A: It is definitely normal to feel confused about dating. One of the basic ideas in dialectical behavior therapy (DBT) is that two seemingly opposite truths can occur at the same time: you can want to date *and* not feel ready. Or, you can feel nervous about dating *and* still take steps toward feeling more comfortable. I would encourage you to take some time to explore your thoughts and feelings some more. A journaling prompt like this one may help:

First, describe the situation. What are all of your choices? Imagine how each of those choices might work out. Tune in to your emotional reaction to each outcome; do you feel excited? Scared? Happy? Guilty? Try to identify what choices bring on mostly positive feelings, and which bring on more negative feelings.

_____

_____

_____

_____

_____

It's also important to keep in mind that there is no rush about making a decision like this one. Take your time in figuring out what's right for you, and when it's right—especially about being physically intimate with someone else. Only you can decide what's best for you. If you ever feel like you are being pressured into something that doesn't feel comfortable to you, please talk to a trusted adult about it right away and skip to the Crisis Resources section (page 123) for additional support.

I HAVE A QUESTION ABOUT STRESS AND . . .

Being in a Relationship

Q: I've been in a relationship for a few months, and we really love each other, but we fight a lot. We have so many ups and downs that I'm not sure it's right for us to stay together. Then again, I can't stand the thought of breaking up. I would feel so heartbroken, and I'm scared I'll never find the same kind of love we have. My mom and my friends are telling me it's not healthy to fight so much, but I just can't figure out my own feelings. How do I decide what to do?

A: I understand exactly what you're saying, and this is a really difficult decision to make. It can help to have other people's opinions on the matter, but you're right—you have to figure out your own thoughts and feelings in order to make a decision that feels right to you. This is one of those times where tuning in to your "wise mind" can be really helpful.

Here's an example:

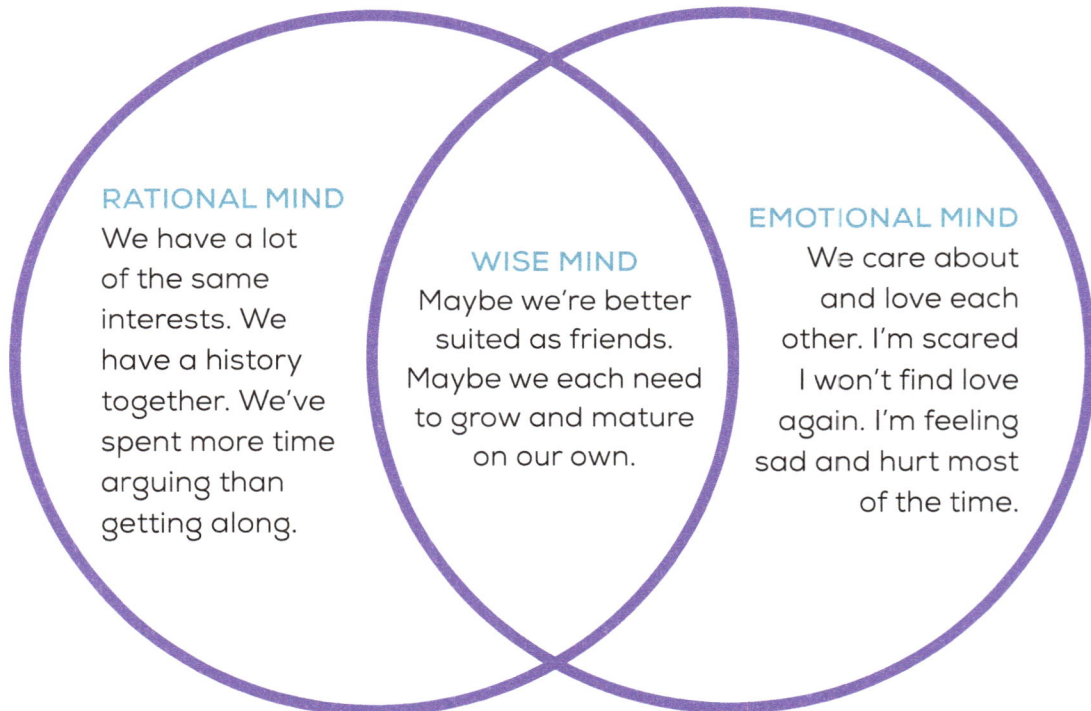

RATIONAL MIND
We have a lot of the same interests. We have a history together. We've spent more time arguing than getting along.

WISE MIND
Maybe we're better suited as friends. Maybe we each need to grow and mature on our own.

EMOTIONAL MIND
We care about and love each other. I'm scared I won't find love again. I'm feeling sad and hurt most of the time.

Now, fill out your own "Wise Mind" diagram. Under Rational Mind, add all the facts about the situation. Under Emotional Mind, add all of your gut feelings.

After filling out as many thoughts and feelings as you can, reflect on your decision. Once you take into account all of the facts and feelings involved, your wise mind should guide you to a more informed decision.

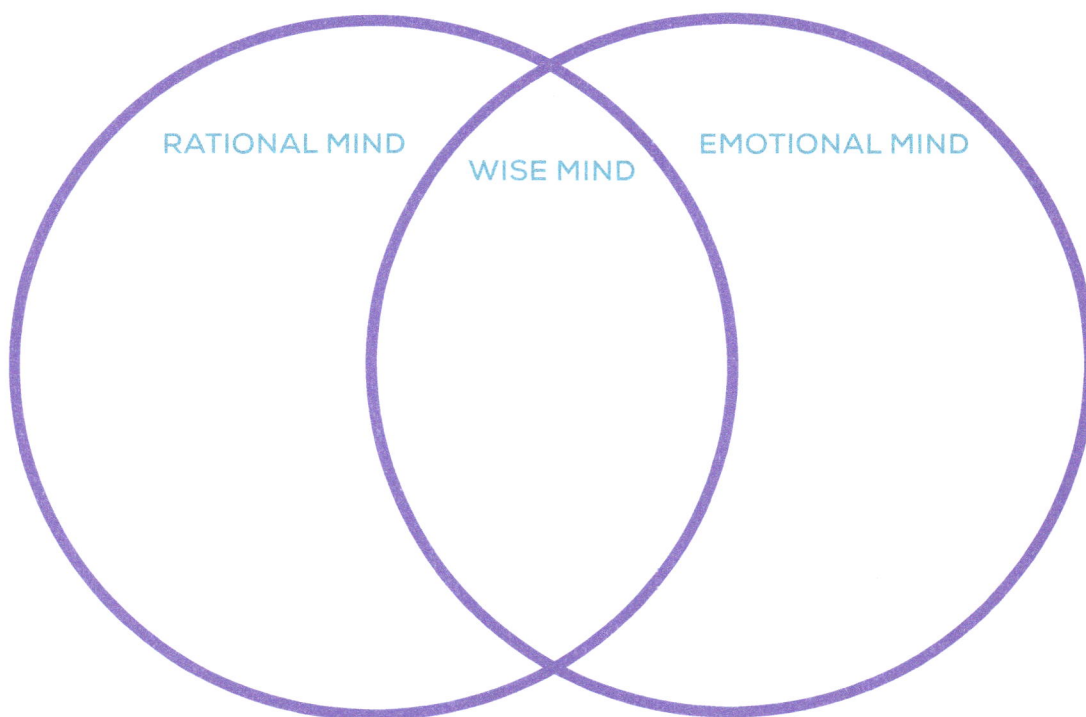

RATIONAL MIND   WISE MIND   EMOTIONAL MIND

I HAVE A QUESTION ABOUT STRESS AND . . .

Using Alcohol and Drugs

Q: I've made the decision to not drink, vape, or use drugs for a couple of reasons. I don't like the feeling of not being in control if I'm drunk or high, and I play sports, so I try to take good care of my body. When I'm out with friends, it feels like more and more people are getting drunk or high, and I feel left out and bored. Sometimes my friends will give me a hard time about it, too, which is annoying and embarrassing. How do I handle that and still keep my friendships?

A: First of all, great job on making such a healthy choice! It can be a hard decision to make, and an even harder one to maintain, especially when your friends have chosen different paths. There might be other ways to connect with your friends that are fun, such as deejaying, dancing, playing video games, or taking pictures. If you've tried all different kinds of things and still feel left out and bored, then I wonder if you'd feel more comfortable socializing with other people. Seek out other friends, classmates, and peers who also abstain from substance use, and see if spending time with them feels more fun and comfortable to you.

Finally, be sure to assert yourself to your closest friends, whose friendships you appreciate the most. Let them know it's important to you that they respect your decision to stay sober, whether they agree with it or not.

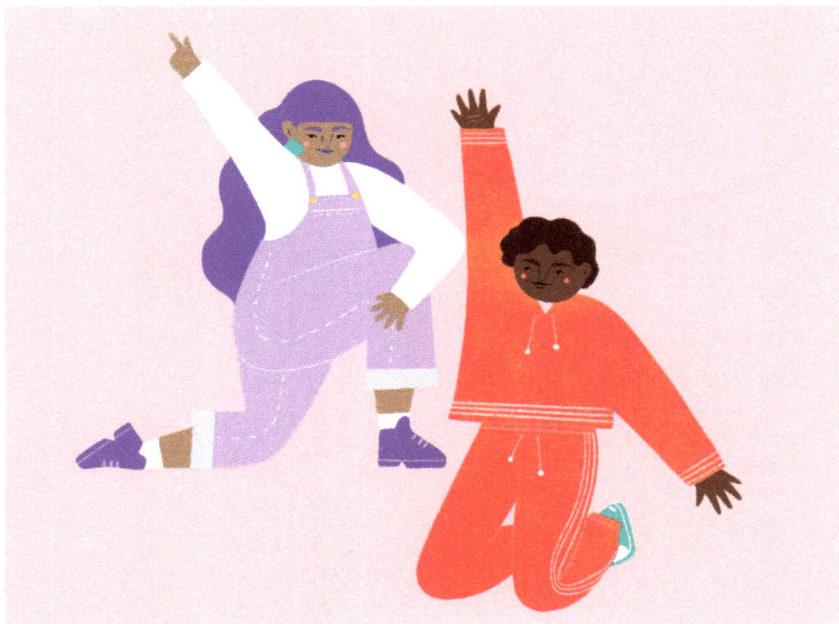

I HAVE A QUESTION ABOUT STRESS AND . . .

Chronic Illness or a Medical Condition

Q: I've always felt different than everyone else because I have a chronic medical condition that not a lot of people understand. When I was younger, I tried to hide it because I felt embarrassed. Now that I'm older, my friends are starting to ask why I miss so much school and why I take medication. I just wish I had a normal life, and it stresses me out to try and hide it. What can I do to feel better about myself and accept my illness?

A: I can tell you that just about every teen I've counseled who has a medical condition has gone through these same exact challenges. At this point in your life, it's natural to start to define who you are, especially in comparison to your peers. When something feels different than "the norm," it can be really hard to accept that as part of your identity. As you get older, you will learn that *everyone* has their own challenges to overcome; you are *not* alone.

Your question has a great answer hidden in it—accepting your illness is probably the key to feeling better about the situation. Acceptance and commitment therapy (ACT) would encourage you to accept what you cannot control—the fact that your medical condition is chronic, it interrupts your life, and it makes other people curious. Then, you can start to focus on creating a life that is meaningful and pleasurable *around* your condition. Define what's important to you (things like friendships, hobbies, or developing some independence from your parents) and start taking action steps toward reaching those goals.

One final idea, which you may already be doing, is to seek out other teens with medical conditions. Maybe your doctor or parents can help you find local support groups, or you can search for online communities where other teens are sharing their personal stories. It's so important to know that you are not alone.

I HAVE A QUESTION ABOUT STRESS AND . . .

Being Embarrassed

Q: Last week, something really embarrassing happened to me in front of my entire class. Everyone laughed, and I felt so awkward! I was hoping that everyone would just forget about it, but a couple of days ago someone posted a video of it on social media. I feel so humiliated, and I don't know what to do to survive this.

A: I know this kind of situation can feel devastating. Please know that you are not the first, or the last, teen who has to deal with an embarrassing moment that's amplified by social media. You will definitely survive this. For now, try to take a broader perspective by realizing that social media is just one part of your life. Refocus on all of the other areas, such as your family relationships, your close friendships, your hobbies, and even your schoolwork.

This is also a great time to use cognitive behavioral therapy (CBT) to "catch, check, and correct" the negative thoughts that are running through your mind, such as "My classmates will tease me for the rest of my life about this!" Concentrating on all of your anxiety about what might go wrong isn't helpful, and it isn't an accurate picture of the future, either. A more accurate and helpful thought is, "This will pass. My classmates will start talking about something else soon." In the meantime, you have to be patient, stay calm, and lean on your family and friends who will stick by you no matter what. If possible, it may even help you to find some humor in the situation (I know, that's really hard right now!).

Finally, it can help to think about how to respond to other people's comments (either face-to-face or online). Try a simple one-liner like "Are you still talking about that?" to let them know you are resilient enough to bounce back from this embarrassing moment.

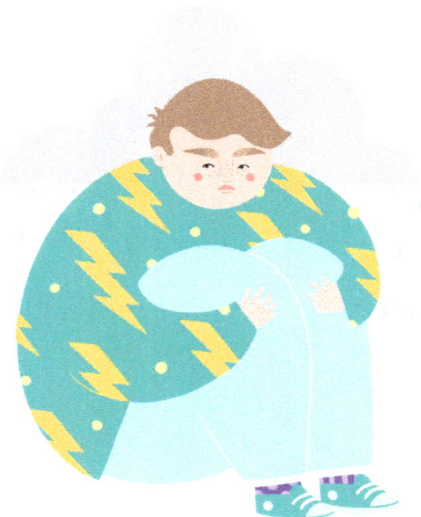

I HAVE A QUESTION ABOUT STRESS AND . . .

Being Bullied

Q: I was bullied when I was younger, and, although it's been a few years, I'm still bothered by it. I can't just "forgive and forget." The hurtful things I heard have really stuck with me. It's been hard for me to build my self-esteem back up. Do you have advice for how I can get over my past?

A: I'm so sorry to hear that you were bullied in the past. Bullying creates an unsafe, insecure, and lonely experience that no one should ever have to go through. It makes a lot of sense that it affected your self-esteem.

It can be very helpful to tell your story. Write it out in a journal, compose letters to the people who bullied you (no need to send them), create a poem or song lyrics, or talk to someone about the details of what you remember. Be sure to focus on the fact that you were not at fault. You were not responsible for the bullying. You did not deserve it.

Next, separate what you cannot control (your past) from what you can control (your future). You are in charge of your thoughts, emotions, and actions. You are in charge of building your self-esteem. Rewrite the story that you started to believe about yourself based on what the bully/bullies said. Focus on what is great about you. What are you good at? What do you like about yourself? What do your friends and family love about you?

Lastly, use your social support system. Bullying causes feelings of loneliness that can keep people isolated for years afterward. Reach out to talk with, hang out with, or even just text friends and family who love you exactly as you are. Accept the love that you deserve!

I HAVE A QUESTION ABOUT STRESS AND . . .

My Parents Fighting

Q: My parents fight all the time. It feels like they argue more often than they get along. They haven't said anything directly to my brother and me, but I've heard them talk about separating, or maybe even getting a divorce. Part of me feels relieved at the thought of no more fighting, but mostly I'm angry, sad, and scared. I'm afraid to say anything to them, because I don't want to make things more stressful than they already are. Should I just keep my feelings to myself?

A: I've spoken with a lot of young people who have lived through this same exact situation. I know it can be very painful, and I'm sorry to hear you are feeling angry, sad, and scared. I can understand your fear of "making things more stressful," but your feelings about the situation are very important, and I imagine your parents would want to support you in any way they can. Think of "walking the middle path," where two seemingly opposite truths coexist: your parents can feel stressed out *and* still be able to love and support you through this.

There are many ways you can practice sharing your feelings, until you feel confident enough to talk with your parents:

- Journaling is a safe and private way to express your feelings. You can use it like a diary; you can write a short story about a teen character living through the same situation; you can write a poem or song; you can draw your feelings; or you can write letters to your parents describing your experience.

- Use a creative outlet like painting, sketching, listening to music, composing your own original music, or taking photos to help you process your feelings.

- Talk with someone you trust. Maybe a caring friend; an aunt, uncle, or grandparent; a teacher, a counselor, a coach, or a religious leader?

- Meditate or pray on it. Set aside a few minutes each day to tune in to your thoughts and feelings about the situation. What sensations do you notice in your body? What emotions arise?

Finally, remember to focus on your own self-care during this difficult time. Take a look back at your self-care wheel from activity 35 (page 82) for specific ideas you can try each day.

I HAVE A QUESTION ABOUT STRESS AND . . .

My Parent(s) Remarrying

Q: My mom is getting remarried, which means my whole life is about to change. My sister and I really like my mom's new partner, but we're moving to a new city, leaving behind our friends, and starting at a new school where we will be "the new kids." My mom has been telling my sister and I that she'll support us any way she can. But I don't see how I'm going to deal with everything changing all at once. What can I do to make this less scary?

A: Wow, that really is a huge change. This situation will definitely require resilience, or the toughness needed to overcome challenges. Take a look back at activity 29: Live It to Learn It (page 72) to review what characteristics you already have that can help you here.

First, focus on gratitude for what you have. It's great that you like your mom's new partner, and it sounds like you can lean on the stability of your relationship with your mom and sister through this uncertain future.

Second, stay connected to your past. Talk with your best friends about how to keep in touch, make an album or video with pictures and memories of your home and school, and maybe ask your family if you can schedule a future visit back.

Third, embrace your future. Being resilient means thinking about how you can make the best out of this situation that you can't control. Talk with your family about what might be the best parts about a new home, a new school, and meeting new people. Write these positive thoughts down, so you can refer back to them when you are feeling scared.

I HAVE A QUESTION ABOUT STRESS AND . . .

My Parents or Family Being Really Strict

Q: My parents have always been really strict, but it seems like it's getting worse as I get older. My curfew is way earlier than everyone else's, and I have an old cell phone, which is super embarrassing. My parents even restrict how much time I can be online at home. I'm missing out on so much and it stresses me out. What can I do to make my parents see me as a responsible teenager who deserves more freedom?

A: I understand how difficult it is to be a teenager with noticeable differences from your friends. I suspect your parents are making these rules to keep you safe (because they love you, of course!). I wonder if they know just how much it bothers you. Have you tried talking with them about it? There's no guarantee that they will change their rules, but it is your right to express yourself to them, especially as you grow older and become more mature and responsible. Here are some tips on how to communicate your needs in a respectful way:

- Collect your thoughts. Exactly what message are you trying to send to your parents? What is important for them to know?

  Example: I'd like my parents to understand how hard it is for me to live with such strict rules. I want them to have more trust in me, and for them to give me the chance to prove that I can make responsible decisions.

- Approach your parents in a calm, open, and direct manner. Ask them when it's a good time to have a conversation. Be ready and willing to share your thoughts and to listen to their side.

- Actively listen. After you've expressed an idea, pay close attention to your parents' response. Pay attention to the message they are trying to express and confirm that you understand them. Use verbal and nonverbal cues to show you are listening.

- Use "I" statements. Focus your statements on your own thoughts, feelings, and experiences, without blaming your parents. For example, instead of saying "You never let me have any fun!" you can say, "I feel sad when I miss out on the fun my friends are having without me."

- Validate. Try your best to understand your parents' thoughts, feelings, and experience. Validation does not mean you have to agree; it simply means that you understand where they are coming from. The more validation you offer to others, the more you will get in return.

I HAVE A QUESTION ABOUT STRESS AND . . .
Getting Along with My Sibling

Q: I'm having a hard time getting along with my sister, who was just diagnosed with a mood disorder. I love her unconditionally, but it can be very hard to deal with her complicated emotions. Everything centers on her. My mom gives her so much time and attention, and it's not fair that I'm left to just handle my problems on my own. I feel angry and resentful toward my sister. How can I feel better about this situation?

A: I can certainly understand how it must feel like everything centers on your sister and her needs right now. I think it's wonderful that you are already tuning in to your feelings and noticing that you feel frustrated, lonely, angry, and resentful. I encourage you to continue expressing your thoughts and feelings as a way to process this. Journal, talk to trusted people outside your family, or use music or art or any creative outlet to express yourself.

I wonder if you've already started to read more about her condition. The more you understand it, the easier it will be for you to make sense of her complicated emotions. This can help you feel more patient, compassionate, and understanding of your sister's and your mom's actions.

Finally, you made a good point about how it's not fair that you are left to handle your problems on your own. While I think it is important for you to practice self-care, and to be mindful that your sister will need urgent attention sometimes, you definitely deserve care from others. Think through these three questions:

Who can offer you the support you need: your mom, another adult in the family, a therapist, a religious leader, or someone else?

_____

_____

_____

_____

_____

_____

What support do you need? More time and attention? Help with solving specific problems? Someone to just listen to you vent?

_____

_____

_____

_____

_____

_____

What might you say to your mom, or another trusted individual, to express that you need this support right now? You might start with, "I understand how important it is to focus on my sister right now, but I'm needing some help processing my own feelings."

_____

_____

_____

_____

_____

_____

I HAVE A QUESTION ABOUT STRESS AND . . .
Family Being Out of Work

Q: A few years ago, I moved in with my extended family. They treat me like their own child, making sure I have everything I need for school, sports, and activities. Recently, my uncle was laid off. He tells me not to worry about it, that he and my aunt will figure it out, but I feel so worried. I think I feel guilty, like I'm an extra burden to them. What can I say or do to help?

A: As a teenager, you are starting to pay more attention to the adult responsibilities happening in your family, things you may not have noticed as a child. It may feel stressful, but it also means you are becoming a more mature and empathetic person. I understand your feeling of guilt, and I wonder if this stems from how deeply you appreciate your family's love and protection these past few years. Don't hesitate to talk with them; that's a wonderful thing to share with them. Ask when would be a good time to talk, and have an honest conversation about what's going on and how you can help.

To be clear, you don't have to carry the same responsibilities as the adults in your family. However, there are plenty of ways you can contribute. Brainstorm about specific ways you can help. Maybe you can pick up extra chores around the house, take care of your cousins, or somehow create time and space for your uncle and aunt to handle their responsibilities. Additionally, you may be able to think of ways to make money last longer, such as coming up with at-home entertainment ideas or helping cook budget-friendly homemade meals instead of eating out.

The key to weathering this storm is to work together as a family!

I HAVE A QUESTION ABOUT STRESS AND . . .

Puberty

Q: I've noticed a lot of changes to my body over the past year, and it makes me feel really uncomfortable. My doctor said this is all a normal part of puberty, but I can't help feeling awkward and self-conscious. I don't have any confidence anymore, and I'm afraid I'm never going to be attractive to other people.

A: Puberty isn't easy—it's a huge amount of change in a short amount of time. But the good news is it's just a phase. First, I encourage you to learn as much as you can about the changes happening to you. Read articles from reliable websites (like those listed in the Resources for Teens section on pages 122–123) and talk more with your doctor, a trusted adult, or an older sibling or cousin. You might even talk to a friend who is feeling the same way! The more you know, the better prepared you are for changes as they arise.

Meanwhile, try to find ways to practice gratitude for your body just as it is. Don't just focus on looks but consider all of the amazing things that you can do and experience with your body—dancing, feeling a warm breeze on your face, tasting something delicious, hugging someone you love. Shift your attention to hobbies and activities (old or new) that make you feel good about yourself. Use your skills and abilities to give back to your community, which can help you gain a new perspective and boost your self-esteem. Look back to your self-care wheel (page 82) for more ideas.

Keep in mind, your personality and your character traits are the real building blocks of self-confidence and the qualities that make you more attractive to others. If you work on taking care of your whole self, then it will be much easier to feel comfortable with your body just as it is.

I HAVE A QUESTION ABOUT STRESS AND . . .

The Future

Q: Sometimes I think about the future and feel a rush of stress. It seems like everyone else has it figured out, but I have no idea how things will work out for me. I'm not sure about college, or what kind of career I want. I just feel lost. How do I figure out some answers?

A: I can assure you, you are not the only one who feels stressed out about the future. In fact, I would say most teens feel the same way! I know it seems like everyone else has it figured out, but that's not quite true. Figuring out and pursuing what you want in your life is rarely a simple path; more often than not, it's a journey with twists and turns. It's completely normal at your age to spend a few years experiencing new and different things in order to map out your unique path forward. Along the way, you will find things that are going to excite and motivate you as you grow.

Look back at activity 27: Challenging My "Worst-Case Worry" (page 69). It's likely that your uncertainty is getting in the way of optimism and excitement about opportunities that lie ahead.

Try to think of college courses in new subjects, trying new jobs, new hobbies, and meeting new people as parts of your journey. These learning experiences can help you define what you like, what you are good at, and what you can contribute to the world. Also, don't be afraid to talk to others about this stressor; you're probably going to find others who feel the same way.

I HAVE A QUESTION ABOUT STRESS AND . . .

Losing Older Relatives or Family Members

Q: I'm very close with my grandmother, who is getting older, and I can tell she feels more tired than ever before. She's in pretty good health, but I can't stop worrying about her. I can't imagine my life without her in it; I would feel so alone. My family members are supportive, but I just can't stop these anxious thoughts from popping up in my head. What can I do to control my worrying about this?

A: You're right—the loss of a loved one, especially one who is so special, can change everything. It is heartbreaking, lonesome, and painful. It is also something you will survive. I think there are two things to focus on in this situation.

First, "thought-stopping" strategies are helpful for controlling these anxious thoughts when they pop up. This might be distraction, such as diving into a creative outlet like music or art, or using mediation and relaxation techniques.

Secondly, try to separate parts of this situation that are out of your control from parts that are in your control. Right now, you still have your grandmother in your life. Take advantage of this time. Try out some, or all, of these ideas:

Tell her what you want her to know. Say "I love you" and "thank you" and anything else in your heart. Jot down some things you want to share here:

_____

_____

_____

_____

_____

_____

_____

_____

_____

Create new memories that you can hold on to for the rest of your life and take pictures and videos. Jot down some ideas for creating new memories:

_____

_____

_____

_____

_____

_____

_____

Consider making a record of your loved one's life. This might include stories in her own words, her favorite recipes, her favorite music, and even advice from her to your future self. Jot down some ideas that you can include in the record:

_____

_____

_____

_____

_____

_____

_____

In these ways, you'll be keeping a part of your grandmother with you forever.

I HAVE A QUESTION ABOUT STRESS AND . . .

Things That I Can't Control

Q: Lately, I've felt stressed out by things that are totally out of my control. I'm talking about big world issues like climate change and racism. I try to avoid the news, but I constantly see political posts on social media, which brings on a panicky feeling. There are a couple of clubs at my school focused on social justice and environmental advocacy, but then I think, what difference can one person make?

A: I know a lot of teens who are affected by these same exact stressors. Environmental and political issues are likely high on your list of personal values, as we explored in activity 16: Defining Your Values (page 52). If you remember, this is part of acceptance and commitment therapy (ACT), which encourages us to accept what we cannot control, define what is meaningful to us, and commit to action to improve our lives in a way that upholds these values.

A little bit of cognitive behavioral therapy (CBT) can also be helpful in examining your thoughts, as we learned about in activity 25: Noticing My Common Thinking Mistakes (page 67). Watch out for all-or-nothing thinking, which might sound like, "I have to make a huge difference in the world, or it's not worth it at all," and replace that with more empowering thinking like "Even small actions can add up to real change."

Moreover, you are not alone in this, and it can help alleviate stress to think of creating strength in numbers. If you team up with others who hold your same values and passions, now you've got some power to effect real change. I would encourage you to at least check out a meeting or two of those clubs or other community organizations. I bet the simple act of showing up, learning more, and meeting others who care about these issues can bring you some hope. And who knows what other opportunities might open up for you to make a real difference?

Write down the one issue that feels most important to you right now, along with next steps you can commit to:

The issue I care most about is:

_____

_____

_____

_____

_____

_____

_____

_____

And I can try these three things to find out more about taking action:

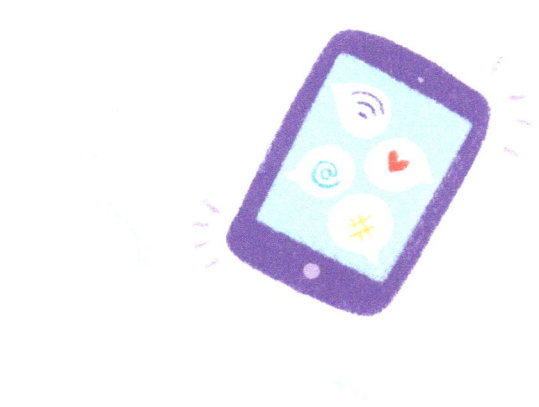

_____

_____

_____

_____

_____

_____

_____

_____

YOU'VE REACHED THE FINISH LINE!

Congratulations! You've made it to the end of this workbook. Let's take a moment to reflect on your experience here at the finish line as compared to the starting line.

Think back to when you started this workbook. What made you decide to start reading? Look back at the first activity on page 27. How were you feeling then?

_____

_____

_____

_____

_____

_____

_____

How are you feeling now, specifically about your ability to conquer stress? Do you have new skills? Do you feel more confident about taking good care of yourself?

_____

_____

_____

_____

_____

_____

_____

Are there any other unanswered questions you still have that you'd like to follow up on by reading on your own, or talking to a parent, therapist, or doctor?

_____

_____

_____

_____

_____

_____

_____

_____

Your Next Steps

You've come so far!

In part 1, you learned all about what stress is, and how it affects your body and mind. You were introduced to 10 stress-reducing techniques that you can incorporate into your daily life, such as deep breathing, mindfulness, progressive relaxation, and visualization. Part 2 focused on many methods of self-care for both physical health and emotional health, and taught you some basic therapy techniques about communicating your needs to others, replacing negative thinking with more positive thinking, and using your "wise mind" to solve problems in a way that balances fact and feeling. Finally, part 3 gave examples of how teens just like you can use this workbook's techniques to manage common stressors.

The themes and strategies covered in this workbook are meant to help you conquer small everyday stressors and to build up your resilience for more intensely stressful times. You can always return to these activities to refresh your skills or try a new strategy. Stress management is a lifelong practice, and we are always learning new ways to invite peace and relaxation into our lives.

For now, take time to celebrate your accomplishment on reaching the end of this workbook. You've worked hard, and you should feel proud of yourself. Now, your next steps will be filled with the knowledge, skills, and confidence you need to live a less stressed, more peaceful life. Enjoy!

Resources for Teens

SOCIAL MEDIA ACCOUNTS

@brenebrown is the Instagram account of Professor Brené Brown, who studies vulnerability, empathy, shame, and courage.

MOBILE APPS

Breathe2Relax is an easy-to-use mobile app designed by the National Center for Telehealth & Technology to teach breathing techniques to manage stress.

Happify is a self-guided app that offers science-based exercises and games to increase positive emotions and reduce worry.

Headspace is a mobile app that guides users through meditation exercises designed to reduce anxiety and stress. Other "modes" offer breathing exercises that guide relaxation, "sleepcasts" that promote sleep, and even lo-fi music that focuses attention.

Mindshift CBT is a free self-guided app that offers a variety of tools based on cognitive behavioral therapy to help reduce anxiety.

Sanvello is a self-guided app with a free version targeting anxiety, stress, and mood disorders through various therapeutic techniques such as deep breathing exercises, daily mood tracking, and identifying negative thinking patterns. It also offers a peer support feature and virtual coaching.

WEBSITES

The Center for Parent and Teen Communication (ParentAndTeen.com) at the Children's Hospital of Philadelphia has resources dedicated to teens, and teens can build a personal, interactive stress management plan.

The Center for Young Women's Health (YoungWomensHealth.org) and **Young Men's Health** (YoungMensHealthSite.org) from Boston Children's Hospital are websites featuring articles on teen health, nutrition and fitness, sexual health, and emotional health.

Go Ask Alice (GoAskAlice.columbia.edu) is a project of Columbia University that offers quizzes and Q&As about typical teen concerns related to health, alcohol and drug use, nutrition, relationships and sexual health, and emotional health.

The Pacer Center's Teens Against Bullying (PacerTeensAgainstBullying.org) is a website created by and for teens, focused on ways that middle school and high school students can address bullying.

Supporting Our Valued Adolescents (SOVA.pitt.edu) is a community blogging project from the University of Pittsburgh, where teens can read articles, share Instagram posts, and contribute their own stories.

Teen Mental Health (TeenMentalHealth.org) uses its website and social media accounts to promote mental health literacy among teens and their families.

TeensHealth from Nemours (TeensHealth.org) offers multiple resources on physical and emotional health, including a stress and coping section.

That's Not Cool (ThatsNotCool.com) is an online social hub focused on creating healthy relationships and preventing interpersonal abuse.

CRISIS RESOURCES

The National Suicide Prevention Lifeline, 1-800-273-8255 (TALK), is available 24/7 for immediate, free, and confidential support for anyone in crisis. Also offers live online chat and a blog at YouMatter.suicidepreventionlifeline.org.

The Trevor Project is an online resource for LGBTQ+ youth, featuring a 24/7 crisis support lifeline at 1-866-488-7386, live online chat, and a text option at 678-678, as well as links to an online LGBTQ+ peer support community at TheTrevorProject.org.

Resources for Parents

BOOKS

How to Talk So Teens Will Listen and Listen So Teens Will Talk by Adele Faber and Elaine Mazlish. This bestselling book is a great read for parents wishing to enhance communication and connection with their teens.

Parenting the New Teen in the Age of Anxiety: A Complete Guide to Your Child's Stressed, Depressed, Expanded, Amazing Adolescence by John Duffy. Written by a clinical psychologist and father, this book offers advice for parents raising adolescents surrounded by a world of access to the internet and social media, and associated increased pressures and stress.

The Teenage Brain: A Neuroscientist's Survival Guide to Raising Adolescents and Young Adults by Frances E. Jensen. Written by a neurologist, this book gives parents insight and practical suggestions for raising adolescents based on their stage of brain development.

PODCASTS

Parenting Great Kids with Dr. Meg Meeker, hosted by a pediatrician and mother, covers relevant topics such as social media, sexual health, and blended families.

Your Teen with Sue and Steph, hosted by the cofounders of Your Teen Media, features interviews with experts on topics like middle school and college admissions.

OTHER RESOURCES

The Center for Parent and Teen Communication (ParentAndTeen.com) at the Children's Hospital of Philadelphia has pages on its website dedicated to parenting tips on building stronger family relationships.

The Center for Young Women's Health (YoungWomensHealth.org) and **Young Men's Health** (YoungMensHealthSite.org) from Boston Children's Hospital are websites featuring articles on teen health, nutrition and fitness, sexual health, and emotional health.

The Greater Good Science Center at UC Berkeley's online magazine, podcast, and online classes, which are intended to promcte "a happier life and a more compassionate society," include insights on parenting.

TeensHealth from Nemours (TeensHealth.org) offers multiple resources on physical and emotional health, including a stress and coping section.

The Verywell family of websites, including **Verywell Health**, **Verywell Fit**, **Verywell Family**, and **Verywell Mind**, is an online resource for information about physical and mental health written by experts including physicians, therapists, and social workers.

Your Teen Media's website and magazine feature a variety of information and resources about raising teenagers.

References

Beck Institute. "What Is Cognitive Behavior Therapy (CBT)?" Accessed September 29, 2020. BeckInstitute.org/get-informed/what-is-cognitive-therapy.

Hayes, Steven. "Acceptance & Commitment Therapy (ACT)." Association for Contextual Behavioral Science. Accessed September 29, 2020. ContextualScience.org/act.

Rathus, Jill H., and Alec L. Miller. *DBT Skills Manual for Adolescents*. New York: Guilford Press, 2014.

Saakvitne, Karen W., and Laurie Anne Pearlman. *Transforming the Pain: A Workbook on Vicarious Traumatization*. New York: W. W. Norton & Company, 1996. See esp. "Self-Care Assessment Worksheet."

Index

Acknowledgments

I would like to first thank Callisto Media for the opportunity to offer teens such critical information about self-care and stress management. I feel exceptionally fortunate to work with teenagers and young adults, whose individuality and courage never cease to inspire me. In turn, I hope this book inspires others with the same resilience and tenacity I've learned from my clients over the years. I am grateful for the life lessons.

I would not be where I am, personally or professionally, without my extraordinary parents, sisters, and Gramma Lola. They loved and supported me through the stress of my teen years, seemingly endless educational pursuits, and countless relocations. The foundation of our family has afforded me the steady hand I offer others.

I'd also like to thank my teachers and mentors throughout graduate school, internships, and fellowships for taking the time to support me, especially when the stress felt insurmountable.

Finally, I am eternally grateful to my husband, whose unconditional love and support are rare and precious, and to our daughter, who shines a light of joy and hope into this world.

About the Author

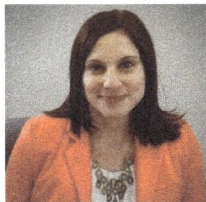

Dr. Carla Cirilli Andrews, PsyD, is a licensed clinical psychologist specializing in teens and young adults. Currently, she maintains a private practice in New Jersey, where she lives with her husband and daughter. Dr. Andrews earned her doctoral degree at the Philadelphia College of Osteopathic Medicine and then completed her fellowship at Yale University's Child Study Center, where she specialized in pediatric psychology. Between her work in the community, hospital, and private practice settings, Dr. Andrews has counseled hundreds of teens and their families on common stress-related issues.